OSCE in Otorhinolaryngology
(Ear, Nose and Throat)

OSCE in Otorhinolaryngology
(Ear, Nose and Throat)

As per the Competency-based Medical Education Curriculum (NMC)

Sumanta Kumar Dutta
MBBS (Gold Medalist) MS ENT (Gold Medalist) DNB ORL
Professor and Head
Department of ENT and Head-Neck Surgery
Nil Ratan Sircar Medical College
Kolkata, West Bengal, India

Sanchari Nandi
MBBS (Gold Medalist) MS ENT (AIIMS, Jodhpur)
Senior Resident
Department of ENT and Head-Neck Surgery
Nil Ratan Sircar Medical College
Kolkata, West Bengal, India

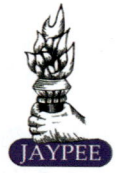

JAYPEE BROTHERS MEDICAL PUBLISHERS
The Health Sciences Publisher
New Delhi | London

Jaypee Brothers Medical Publishers (P) Ltd

Headquarters
Jaypee Brothers Medical Publishers (P) Ltd
EMCA House, 23/23-B
Ansari Road, Daryaganj
New Delhi 110 002, India
Landline: +91-11-23272143, +91-11-23272703
+91-11-23282021, +91-11-23245672
Email: jaypee@jaypeebrothers.com

Corporate Office
Jaypee Brothers Medical Publishers (P) Ltd
4838/24, Ansari Road, Daryaganj
New Delhi 110 002, India
Phone: +91-11-43574357
Fax: +91-11-43574314
Email: jaypee@jaypeebrothers.com

Overseas Office
J.P. Medical Ltd
83 Victoria Street, London
SW1H 0HW (UK)
Phone: +44 20 3170 8910
Fax: +44 (0)20 3008 6180
Email: info@jpmedpub.com

Website: www.jaypeebrothers.com
Website: www.jaypeedigital.com

© 2023, Jaypee Brothers Medical Publishers

The views and opinions expressed in this book are solely those of the original contributor(s)/author(s) and do not necessarily represent those of editor(s) and Publisher of the book.

All rights reserved. No part of this publication may be reproduced, stored or transmitted in any form or by any means, electronic, mechanical, photocopying, recording or otherwise, without the prior permission in writing of the publishers.

All brand names and product names used in this book are trade names, service marks, trademarks or registered trademarks of their respective owners. The publisher is not associated with any product or vendor mentioned in this book.

Medical knowledge and practice change constantly. This book is designed to provide accurate, authoritative information about the subject matter in question. However, readers are advised to check the most current information available on procedures included and check information from the manufacturer of each product to be administered, to verify the recommended dose, formula, method and duration of administration, adverse effects and contraindications. It is the responsibility of the practitioner to take all appropriate safety precautions. Neither the publisher nor the author(s)/editor(s) assume any liability for any injury and/or damage to persons or property arising from or related to use of material in this book.

This book is sold on the understanding that the publisher is not engaged in providing professional medical services. If such advice or services are required, the services of a competent medical professional should be sought.

Every effort has been made where necessary to contact holders of copyright to obtain permission to reproduce copyright material. If any have been inadvertently overlooked, the publisher will be pleased to make the necessary arrangements at the first opportunity.

Inquiries for bulk sales may be solicited at: jaypee@jaypeebrothers.com

OSCE in Otorhinolaryngology (Ear, Nose and Throat)

First Edition: **2023**

ISBN: 978-93-5696-205-7

Printed at: Sterling Graphics Pvt. Ltd.

Dedication

To our beloved students

and

To my parents, my wife Prof (Dr) Baishali Chakraborty and my little angel Kojagori for being the source of strength and support during the preparation of this book.

—**Sumanta Kumar Dutta**

To my family [(my parents—Mrs Sampa and Dr Tapas); Sayantani, Abhishek and Abhay] for their unwavering love and support.

To Dr SK Dutta Sir, for placing his trust in me.

—**Sanchari Nandi**

Preface

It is a great pleasure to introduce our book—*OSCE in Otorhinolaryngology (Ear, Nose and Throat)*, a unique text with Objective Structured Clinical Examination (OSCE)-patterned questions, based on the new CBME undergraduate curriculum for the Indian Medical Graduate.

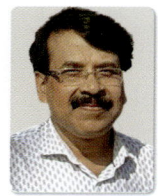

Sumanta Kumar Dutta

The inception of this unique concept arose from the dire need of the hour, after seeing our students struggle with the new concept of OSCE-based questions, which have now become a mandatory part of their curriculum. As we all know, OSCE can be a really scoring section of any examination if the candidate is oriented with the concept and well-prepared beforehand. We realized that there were no resources available, to cater to this specific need of the undergraduates studying for ENT. Hence, it was a dream to help the brilliant young minds get acclimatized to OSCE preparation.

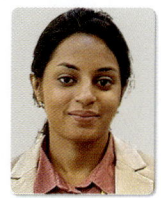

Sanchari Nandi

What makes our book Unique?
Image-based learning, with multiple simple illustrations/diagrams can help students retain important concepts better and finally implement them in their examination. The book is subdivided into 8 major sections with questions given first, followed by the answers at the end of each chapter, for the student to solve and assess their own performance. We intend to spark an interest in the mind of any student (undergraduate or postgraduate) who picks up this book as well as sensitize them to the advancement that has taken place in the field of ENT. It should be noted that this book is an additional resource to your textbook and not an alternative to it.

Bringing this book to life was a thoroughly enjoyable and challenging experience given the limited time we had. We urge all our readers to write to us and provide their positive criticism, valuable feedback and suggestions via email (drskduttaentkolkata@gmail.com, nandi.sanchari@gmail.com), for improving the further editions to come.

Read on and Enjoy!

Sumanta Kumar Dutta
Sanchari Nandi
March, 2023

Acknowledgments

- ❖ We take this opportunity to extend our deep sense of reverence to everyone who has helped us in this endeavor.
- ❖ We thank all the Faculties and Residents of NRS Medical College (Kolkata) for their overwhelming support and constant cooperation in bringing this project to fruition.
- ❖ We express our gratitude to Dr Anupam Roy and Dr Indranil Khatua for their contributions to the 'Throat and Neck' sections.
- ❖ We thank Dr Tapas Kumar Nandi for his contributions to the 'Ear and Throat' sections.
- ❖ Special thanks to Dr Uddeepta Dutta for his contributions to the 'Oral Cavity' chapter.
- ❖ Our sincere thanks to Prof (Dr) Sri Krishna Mondal for his valuable contributions to the 'Recent Advances' section.
- ❖ Special thanks to our beloved residents, Dr Md Nadeem Hasan and Dr Veeus Nag Mukherjee for their immense help with the photographs.
- ❖ Special thanks to Mr Asis Kumar Sinha for helping us format the manuscript and take photographs for the 'Clinical Methods' sections of the book.
- ❖ We are immensely grateful to Prof (Dr) Baishali Chakraborty for taking out time from her busy schedule for proofreading the book.
- ❖ We thank Dr Aditya Tayal [Team Lead–UG Publishing, M/s Jaypee Brothers Medical Publishers (P) Ltd, New Delhi Branch] for his advice and cooperation throughout this project.
- ❖ We sincerely thank Mr Sabyasachi Hazra [Senior Business Manager–Publishing, M/s Jaypee Brothers Medical Publishers (P) Ltd, Kolkata Branch] for his prompt support and guidance, in making this title a reality. This would not have been possible in such short notice without his timely intervention.
- ❖ We thank our support staff, Mr Sanu Roy and Mr Vishal Mallick for volunteering to be our model patients for the examination photographs.
- ❖ We take this opportunity to express our heartfelt gratitude to the Principal, the Medical Superintendent cum Vice-Principal and the administrative authorities of NRS Medical College (Kolkata) for constantly supporting us in the upliftment of our department and fulfilment of our project as and when required.
- ❖ We are grateful to our Patients for consenting to be a part of this book.

Contents

Section 1: Ear

1. Anatomy — 3
2. Physiology — 13
3. Clinical Methods — 19
4. Surgical Procedures — 27
5. Development — 31
6. Audio-Vestibulometry — 37

Section 2: Nose and Paranasal Sinuses

7. Anatomy — 49
8. Physiology — 56
9. Clinical Methods — 59
10. Surgical Procedures — 71
11. Development — 78

Section 3: Throat

12. Oral Cavity — 83
13. Salivary Glands — 93
14. Pharynx and Esophagus — 96
15. Larynx and Trachea — 105

Section 4: Neck

16. Neck Proper — 119
17. Thyroid and Parathyroid Glands — 128

Section 5: Instruments

18. OPD Instruments — 135
19. OT Instruments — 142

Section 6: Imaging

20. X-rays in ENT — 157
21. Miscellaneous Imaging — 169

Section 7: Recent Advances

| 22. Recent Advances | 175 |

Section 8: Skill Assessment Topics

| 23. Skill Assessment Topics | 197 |

Bibliography   *201*
Index   *203*

EAR

Section Outline

1. Anatomy
2. Physiology
3. Clinical Methods
4. Surgical Procedures
5. Development
6. Audio-Vestibulometry

Anatomy

Q1. The external auditory canal (EAC) is divided into two parts—cartilaginous and bony:

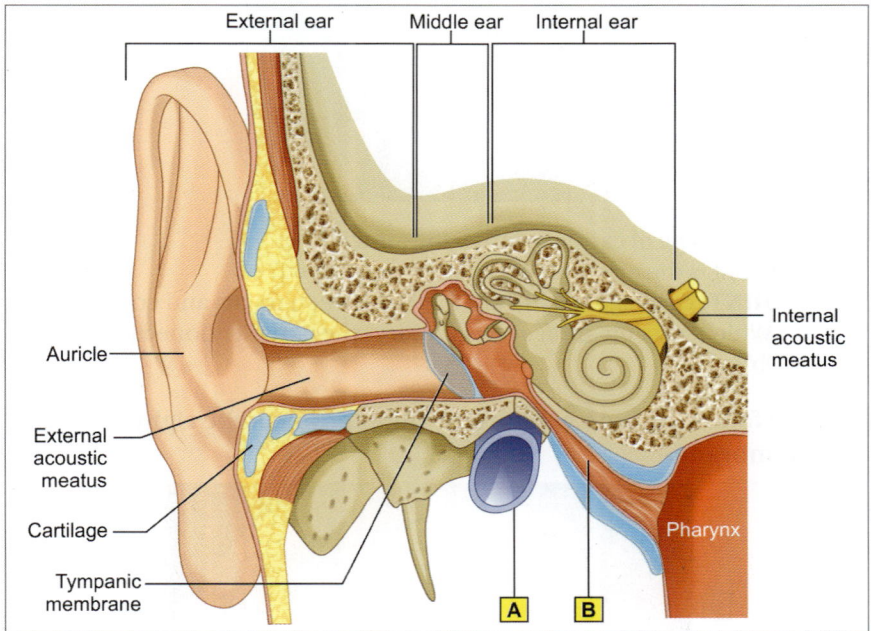

a. Mention the length of each part.
b. What is the deficiency in the bony and cartilaginous EAC known as respectively?
c. What is the clinical significance of these deficiencies?
d. Explain why furunculosis is not seen in the bony EAC?
e. Label the structures 'A' and 'B'.

Q2. Regarding auricle/pinna answer the following:

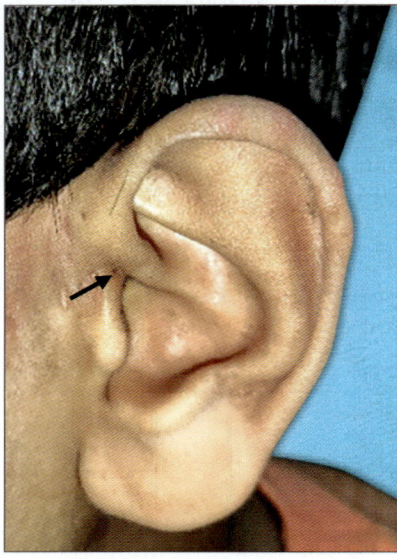

a. What type of cartilage forms the auricle?
b. What is the area marked by the arrow called?
   HINT! cartilage is deficient there (between tragus and crus of helix)
c. Which incision in ear surgery utilizes the part mentioned in question 'b'?

Q3. The following is an endoscopic photograph of the right tympanic membrane.

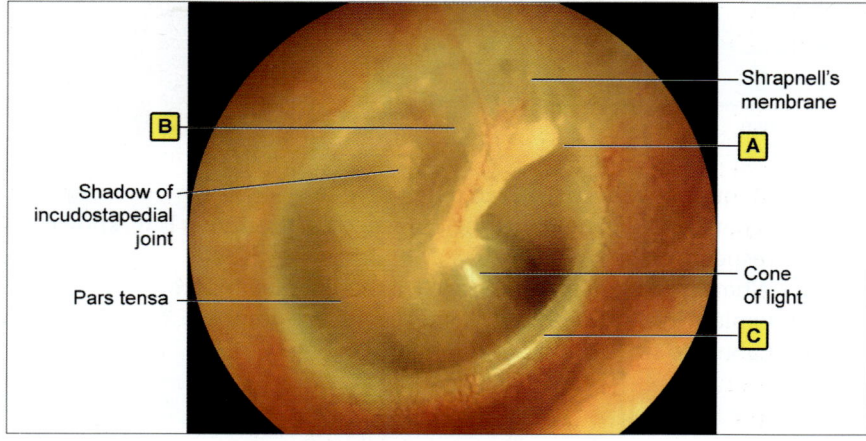

a. Label the structures marked (A), (B) and (C).
b. What is the nerve supply of the anterior and posterior half of the lateral surface of the tympanic membrane?
c. What is Jacobson's nerve?

Q4. The following is showing the coronal section through the external canal and middle ear at the level of the malleus handle.

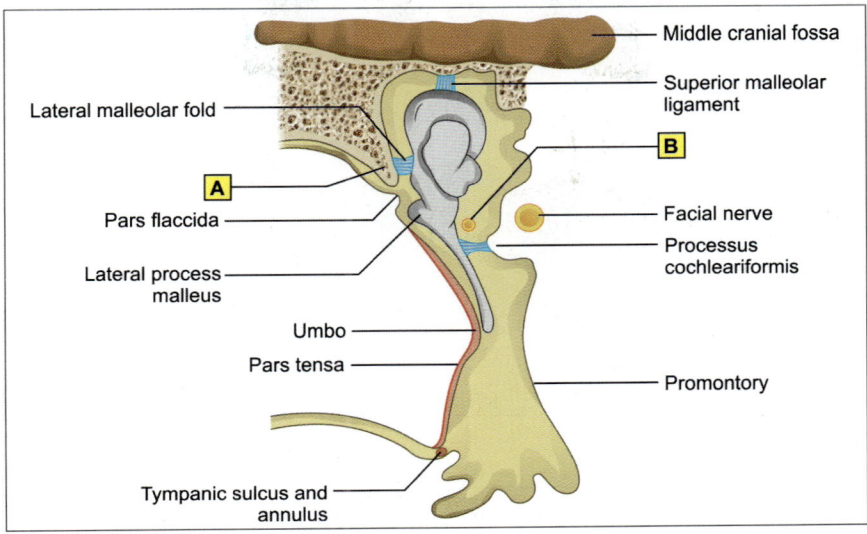

a. Label the structure marked (A). What is the nerve marked as (B)?
b. Mention the three types of fiber arrangements in the middle fibrous layer of the pars tensa.
c. Name one condition in which there is "sagging" of the postero-superior part of the deeper external canal wall.

Q5. The following diagram is showing the nerve supply of the external auditory canal:

a. What is Arnold's nerve?
b. What is the nerve supply of the postero-superior wall of the EAC (marked by double question marks in the figure)?
c. What is the sign for loss of sensation in that part?
d. Name one disease in which lesions are seen in the distribution of the facial nerve.

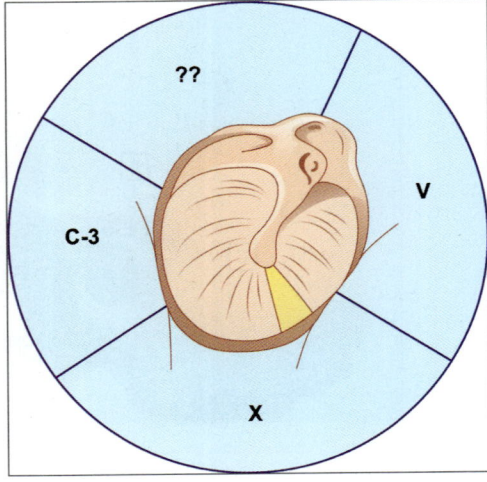

SECTION 1: Ear

Q6. The diagram shows the structures in relation to the middle ear:

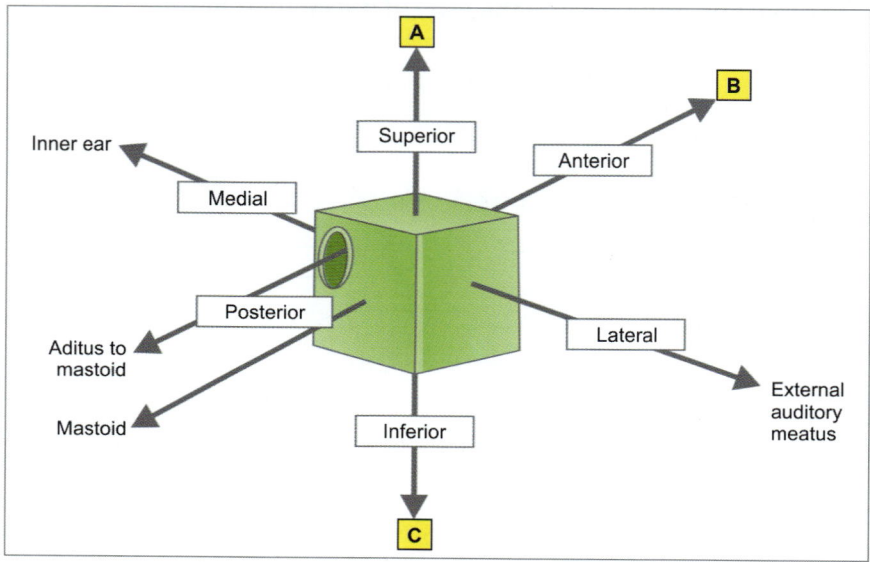

Answer with respect to A, B and C as the following:

A (Two structures in relation to superior wall)	B (Three structures in relation to anterior wall)	C (Two structures in relation to inferior wall)
1.	1.	1.
2.	2.	2.
	3.	

Q7. With relation to the middle ear anatomy, answer the following:

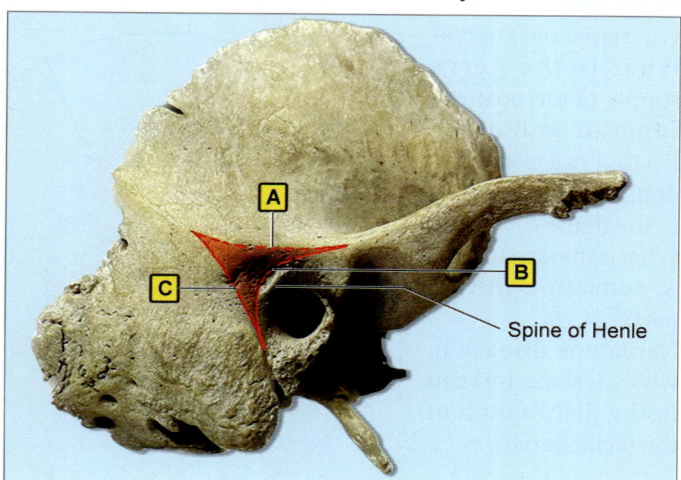

a. What is structure in relation to the protympanum?
b. What is the triangle shaded in red, being shown in the image of the temporal bone below?
c. Label A, B and C marked in the following figure.
d. At what depth is the antrum located?

CHAPTER 1: Anatomy

Q8. The given figure shows the structures in the retrotympanum as seen from the mesotympanum.

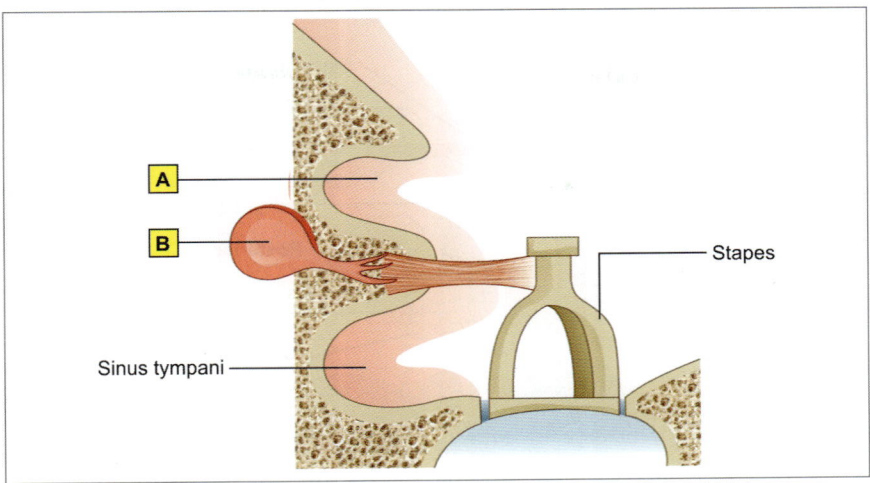

a. Label the structures marked (A) and (B) in the diagram.
b. What are the boundaries of the sinus tympani?
c. Name one intact canal wall mastoidectomy technique in which the area 'A' is accessed.
d. Name one surgical application of the technique asked in 'c'.

Q9. With reference to the anatomy of the labyrinth, observe the diagram and answer the following:

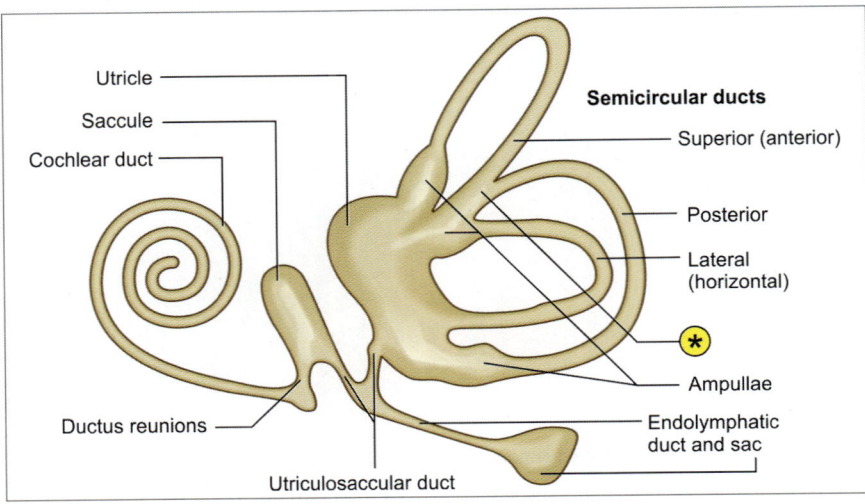

a. How many openings of the semicircular canals are present in the vestibule?
b. How many openings does the vestibule have (in total)?
c. The aqueduct of cochlea connects which two structures?
d. Helicotrema connects which two structures?
e. Label the structure marked with '*'.

Q10. Observe the following diagram showing the stapes in the oval window and its relation with the underlying vestibule:

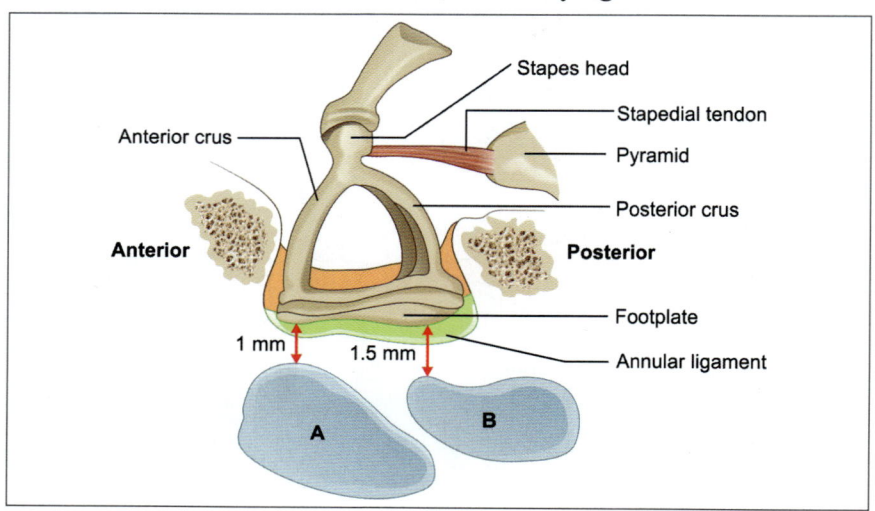

a. What are the structures marked 'A' and 'B'?
b. Name one function of both A and B?
c. What is cochlear otosclerosis?
d. Which structure passes through the aqueduct of vestibule?

Q11. The following image shows anatomy of the inner ear:

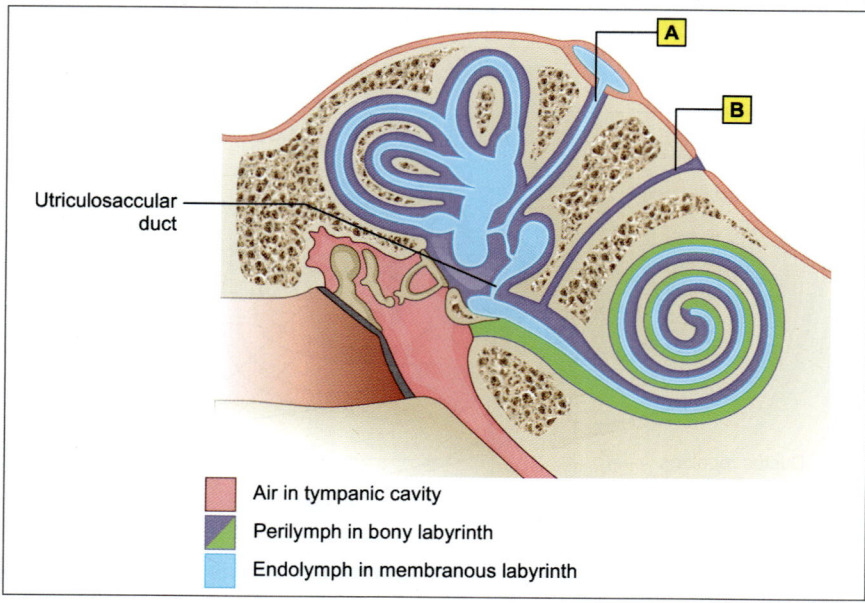

a. Label the structures marked as 'A' and 'B'
b. What is the clinical significance if the structure 'A' is enlarged?

Q12. The following diagram shows the anatomic interrelations at the fundus of the internal auditory canal:

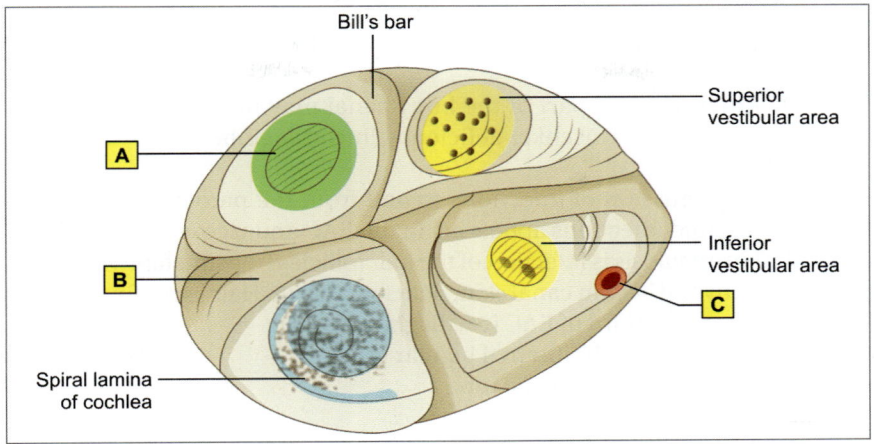

a. Label A, B and C
b. Name three tumors of the cerebellopontine angle.
c. Name a syndrome in which bilateral facial palsy can be seen.

ANSWERS

Ans 1:
   a. Bony EAC–16 mm (inner 2/3rd), cartilaginous EAC–8 mm (outer 1/3rd)
   b. Anteroinferior part of the bony canal may present a deficiency—Foramen of Huschke; deficiency in cartilaginous EAC—Fissure of Santorini
   c. Transmission of infections to and from the parotid or superficial mastoid infections appearing in the EAC and vice versa
   d. Furunculosis is infection of the hair follicles (mostly staphylococcal). Bony EAC—thin canal skin, deficient of hair. Hair is confined to only outer one-third of EAC (cartilaginous part)
   e. 'A': Jugular bulb (internal jugular vein)
      'B': Pharyngotympanic tube

Ans 2:
   a. Elastic fibrocartilage
   b. Incisura terminalis
   c. Lempert's endaural incision

Ans 3:
   a. The parts labelled A, B and C are shown in Figure

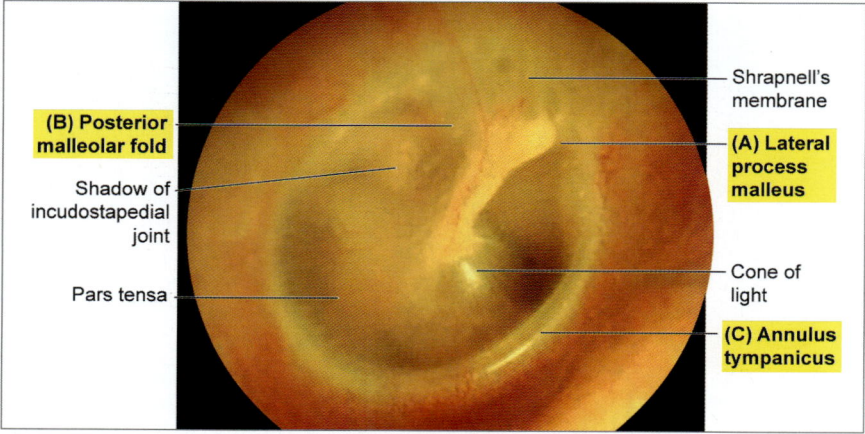

   b. Anterior half of tympanic membrane: Auriculo-temporal nerve (V_3)
      Posterior half of tympanic membrane: Auricular branch of vagus nerve (X)
   c. Jacobson's nerve—tympanic branch of cranial nerve IX

CHAPTER 1: Anatomy

Ans 4:
- a. A: *Scutum* (meaning SHIELD in Latin; also known as—lateral attic wall or outer attic wall)—thin sharp bony spur at the junction of the attic outer wall and the superior wall of the external auditory canal. It is the first bony structure to be eroded by an attic cholesteatoma secondary to a retraction pocket of the pars flaccida
  B: Chorda tympani nerve
- b. Radial, circular and parabolic fibers
- c. Acute mastoiditis

Ans 5:
- a. Auricular branch of vagus (Xth nerve)
- b. Sensory fibers of cranial nerve VIII (supplying through the auricular branch of vagus)
- c. Loss of sensation over the posterior-superior wall of EAC—Hitzelberger's sign (seen in acoustic neuroma)
- d. Herpes zoster oticus

Ans 6:

A (Two structures in relation to superior wall)	B (Three structures in relation to anterior wall)	C (Two structures in relation to inferior wall)
1. Middle cranial fossa	1. Tensor tympani muscle	1. Jugular bulb
2. Temporal lobe	2. Eustachian tube	2. Internal carotid artery
	3. Internal carotid artery	

Ans 7:
- a. Protympanum – portion of middle ear around tympanic orifice of Eustachian tube
- b. MacEwen's (suprameatal) triangle: overlies mastoid antrum, characterized by multiple small perforating vessels and hence known as cribrose (cribriform) area
- c. Figure showing boundaries of **MacEwen's triangle:**
  a—temporal line (superiorly)
  b—postero-superior rim of bony external auditory canal
  c—line drawn as a tangent to the external canal (posteriorly)
- d. 1–1.5 cm deep to the lateral wall forming the MacEwen's triangle

Ans 8:
- a. A. Vertical segment of facial nerve
  B. Facial recess
- b. Boundaries of sinus tympani:
  - Superiorly: Ponticulus
  - Inferiorly: Subiculum
  - Laterally: Vertical segment of facial nerve
- c. Posterior tympanotomy
- d. Cochlear implantation (by posterior tympanotomy technique)

Ans 9:
   a. 5 openings, opening into the postero-superior part of the vestibule. Each canal has an ampullated end, opening independently into the vestibule (i, ii, iii); non-ampullated end of the lateral SCC (iv), non-ampullated ends of the posterior and superior canal join to form crus commune (v) which opens into the vestibule
   b. 7 openings in total (Previous 5 + opening of the endolymphatic duct passing through the aqueduct of vestibule + oval window [closed by the footplate of stapes])
   c. Aqueduct of cochlea connects scala tympani to subarachnoid space
   d. Helicotrema connects scala vestibuli and scala tympani
   e. Crus commune

Ans 10:
   a. 'A': Saccule; 'B': Utricle
   b. Linear acceleration
   c. Involves region of round window or other areas in the otic capsule and may cause sensorineural hearing loss due to liberation of toxins into inner ear fluid
   d. Endolymphatic duct

Ans 11:
   a. 'A'—Aqueduct of vestibule
      'B'—Cochlear aqueduct
   b. Enlarged vestibular aqueduct: Fluctuant, progressive sensorineural hearing loss, generally bilateral

Ans 12:
   a. A: Fallopian canal (VII nerve)
      B: Transverse crest
      C: Singular foramen
   b. Three tumors of the cerebello-pontine angle: i. Acoustic neuroma, ii. Meningioma, iii. Epidermoid (cholesteatoma)
   c. Melkersson syndrome

CHAPTER 2

Physiology

Q1. The following image shows the organ of Corti:

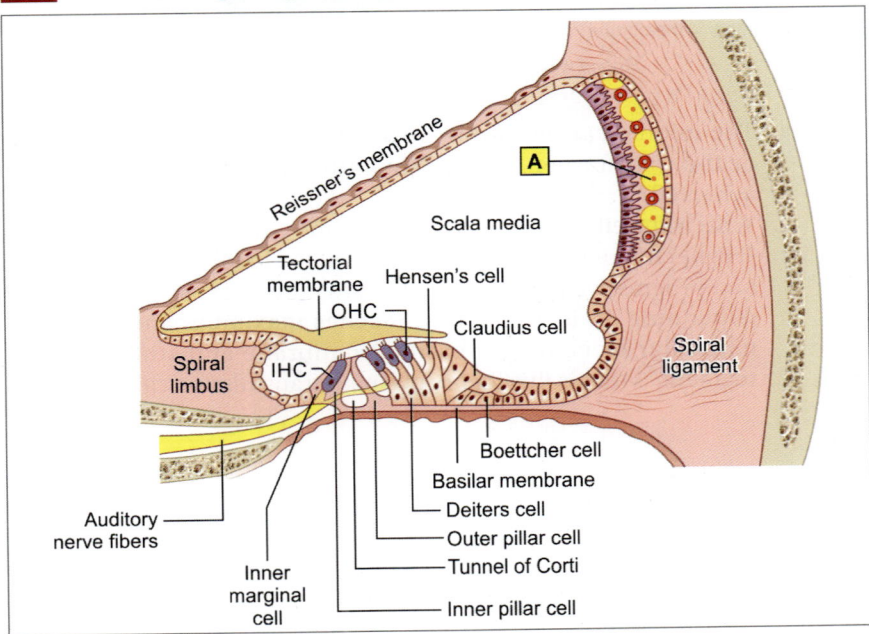

a. What is the structure marked by 'A' in the image above?
b. What is its function?
c. What is the location and area number of the auditory cortex?

Q2. With regard to the transmission of sound, answer the following:

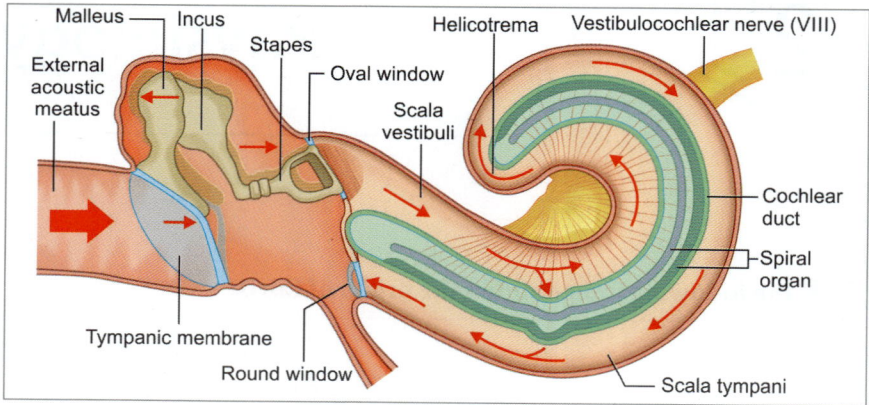

a. The middle ear performs the impedance matching mechanism or the transformer action. What are the 3 points, by which it is achieved?
b. What is the effective vibratory area of the tympanic membrane?
c. "Higher frequencies are represented in the basal turn of the cochlea and progressively lower ones towards the apex. So a sound wave depending on its frequency, reaches maximum amplitude at a particular place on the basilar membrane and stimulates that segment." What is this theory of sound transmission called?

Q3. The following diagram shows the inputs and outputs for the maintenance of the body's equilibrium:

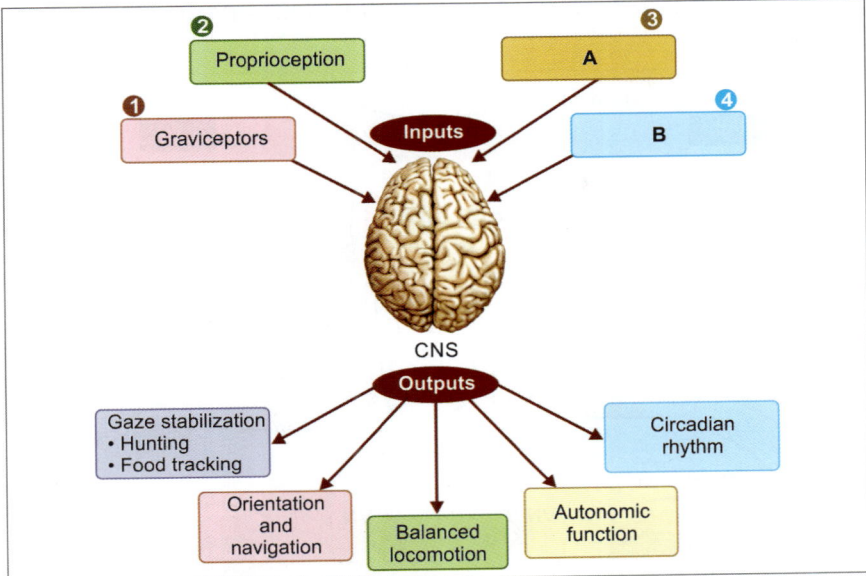

a. What are the two more organs of input marked as 'A' and 'B' which provide important inputs for balance?
b. Utricle and saccule are responsible for what kind of motion?
c. Where are Cristae located? What kind of motion does it detect?

Q4. The following diagram shows a reflex. When the head tilts towards the right, the eyes compensate by moving an equal and opposite degree to the left, in order to maintain stabilization of vision.

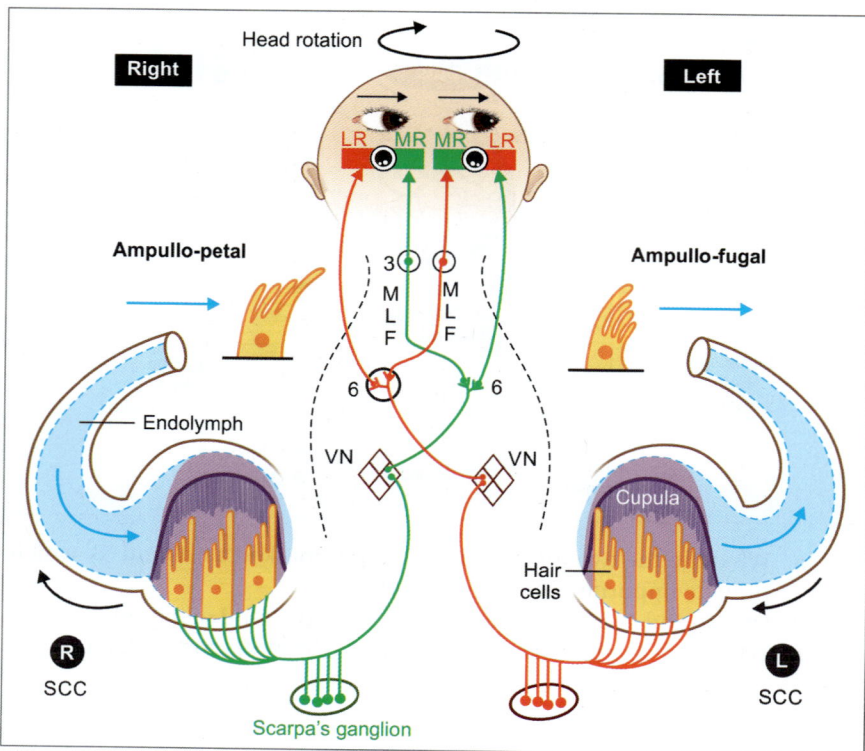

LEGEND: SCC: Semi-circular canal; MR: Medial rectus; LR: Lateral rectus; MLF: Medial longitudinal fasciculus; VN: Vestibular nucleus

a. What is the name of this reflex, responsible for gaze stabilization, being shown?
b. What is the orientation of the superior (vertical) semi-circular canals to the midline?
c. What is the orientation of the lateral semi-circular canals to the horizontal?

CHAPTER 2: Physiology

ANSWERS

Ans 1:
   a. 'A': Stria vascularis
   b. Pivotal role in cochlear homeostasis by generating endo-cochlear potential and maintaining the unique ion composition of the endolymph
   The flow of K⁺ occurs from the scala media through hair cells into the perilymphatic spaces as well as through the epithelial gap junction network into the spiral ligament. K⁺ from the spiral ligament is transported via the stria vascularis into the scala media

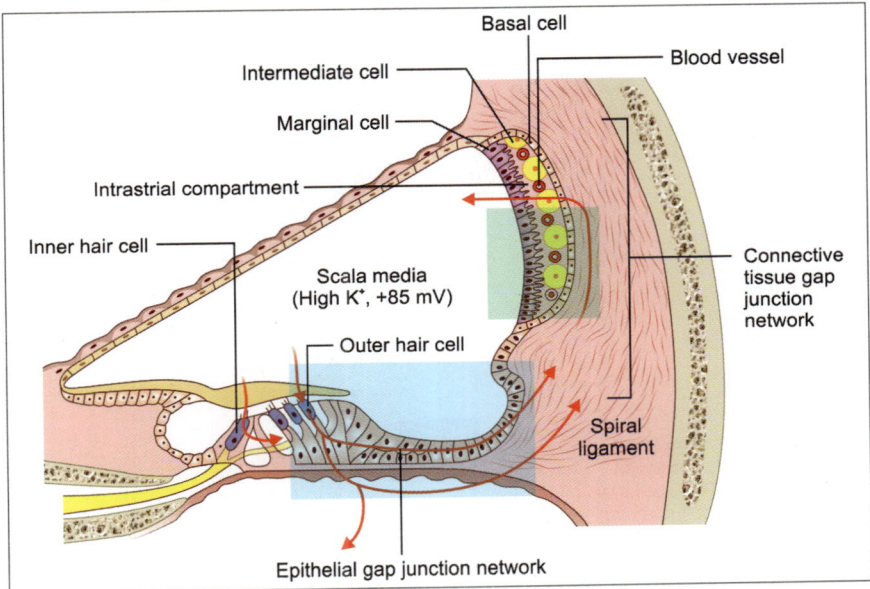

   c. Superior temporal gyrus, Broadmann area 41

Ans 2:
   a. Three points of impedance matching mechanism of ear:
      i. **Area ration:** The major transformer mechanism within the middle ear is the ratio of the tympanic membrane area to the stapes footplate area (the area ratio). The tympanic membrane gathers force over its entire surface and then couples the gathered force to the smaller footplate of the stapes. The human tympanic has an area that is 20 times larger than that of the stapes footplate
      ii. **Ossicular lever action:** The rotating malleus is 1.3 times longer than the incus arm
      iii. **Curved membrane effect:** Tympanic membrane moves more at the periphery than at the center where the malleus handle is attached
   b. 55 sq. mm
   c. Travelling wave theory of Von Bekesy

Ans 3:
   a. A: Labyrinth (vestibular organs)
      B: Eyes (vision)
   b. Linear acceleration, deceleration or gravitational pull during head tilts
   c. Cristae: Located in ampullary ends of semi-circular canals. Responsible for angular acceleration

Ans 4:
   a. VOR: Vestibulo-ocular reflex
   b. 45° from the midsagittal plane, as shown below:

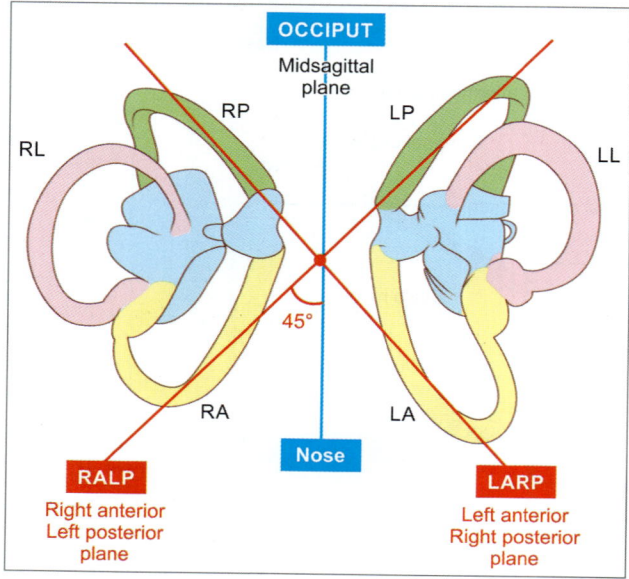

   c. 30° tilted upwards from the horizontal plane at its anterior end

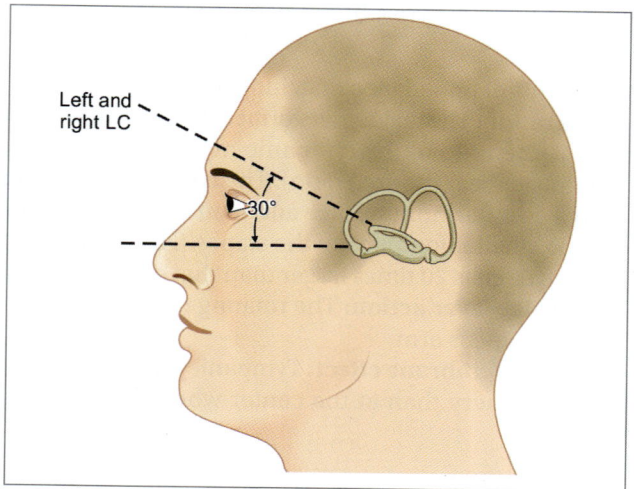

Clinical Methods

Q1. The following image shows a tuning fork test being performed on a patient:

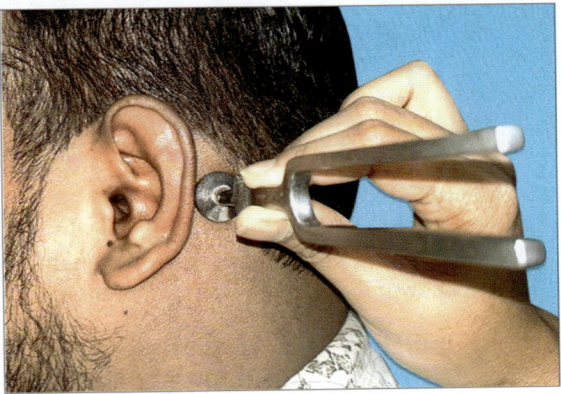

    a. What is being tested in this patient?
    b. Where is the tuning fork placed in this test?

Q2. The following image shows the procedure of making a mop for removing discharge or debris from the ear canal:

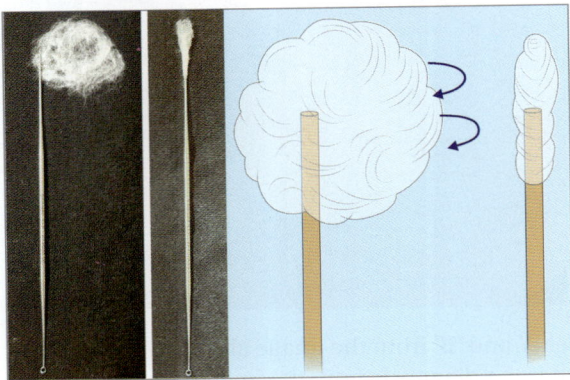

    a. What is the precaution that should be taken while making this mop? (**HINT!**...Answer lies in the image!!)
    b. What treatment should you do for traumatic rupture of the tympanic membrane.

Q3. A 17-year-old boy came with the complaint of decreased hearing to the ENT OPD. The following examination was done:

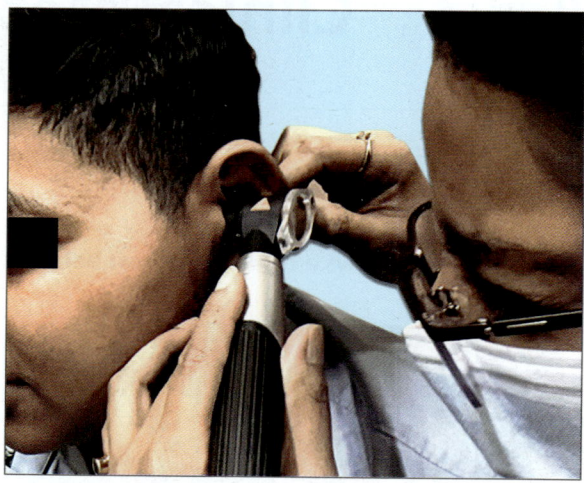

a. What is the procedure being performed?
b. How is the pinna held for performing this test?
c. What should be checked for before performing this test?
   (**HINT!** The answer lies in checking some tenderness....)

Q4. The following image is of a 30-year-old man with history of recurrent ear discharge from childhood:

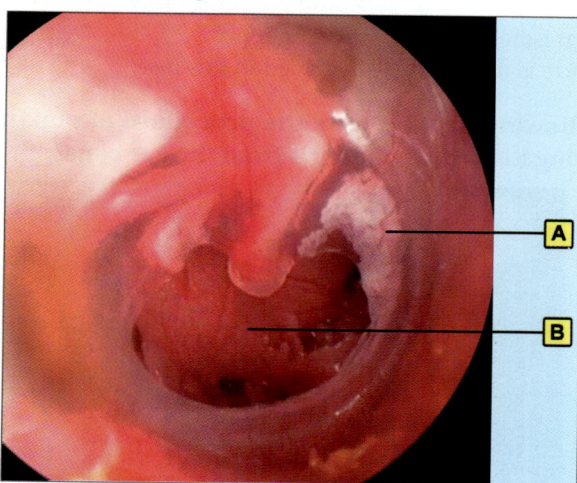

a. Label 'A' and 'B' from the image above.
b. What is the diagnosis from the image shown above?
c. What is a central perforation?

Q5. This is the tympanic membrane photo of a 6-year-old girl having acute pain in the right ear following an episode of fever with URI:

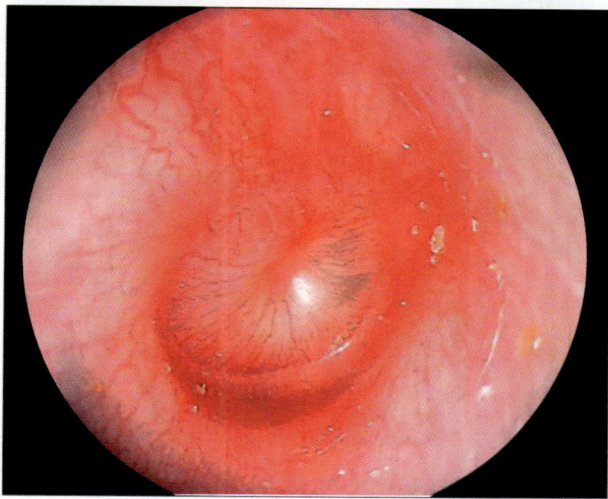

a. What is your diagnosis? Mention the sign.
b. What are the most common organisms responsible for it?

Q6. The following is the tympanic membrane photograph of a 35-year-old male patient with complaint of decreased hearing:

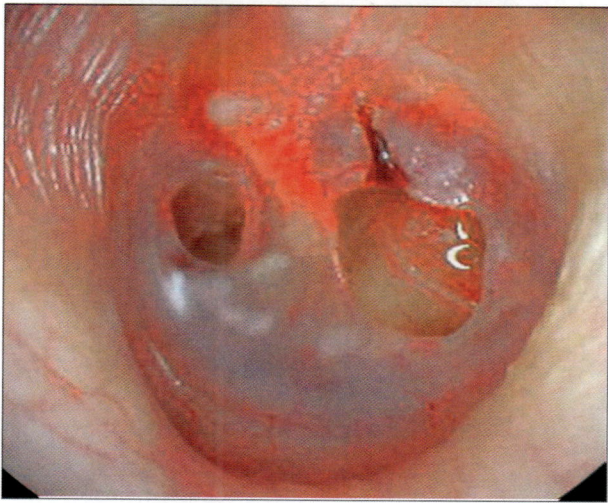

a. What is your diagnosis from this image?
b. There is earache associated with this condition: True/False?
c. What specific treatment will you administer in this patient?

Q7. Observe the photo below:

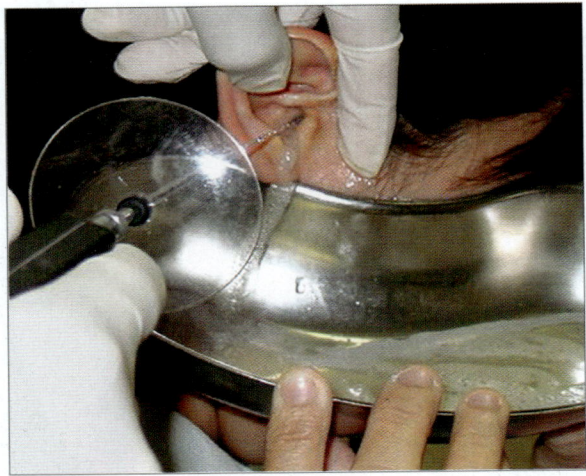

a. What is the procedure being done?
b. What complication can it lead to, after performing?

Q8. The following image shows a patient who developed this condition:

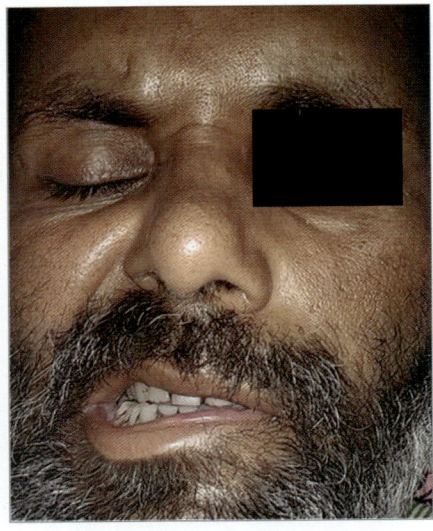

a. What is the condition being shown here?
b. Which is the drug to be given in case the above condition is due to an idiopathic cause?
c. Which is the narrowest segment of the nerve involved in the photo above?

CHAPTER 3: Clinical Methods

Q9. The following is a photograph of a child with earache, ear discharge with fever.

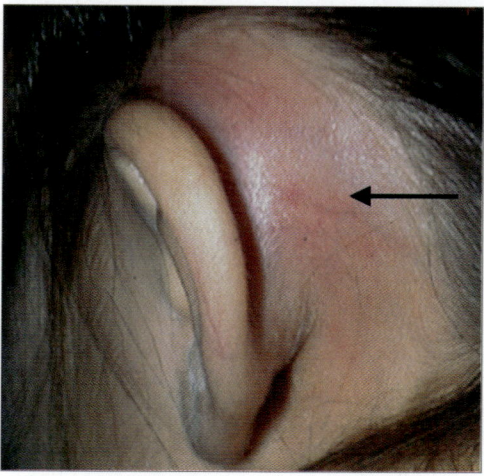

a. What is your diagnosis from the photo?
b. What is battle sign?
c. Name one condition in which the post-aural groove is obliterated.

Q10. In the image below, a test is being performed by applying intermittent pressure on the tragus:

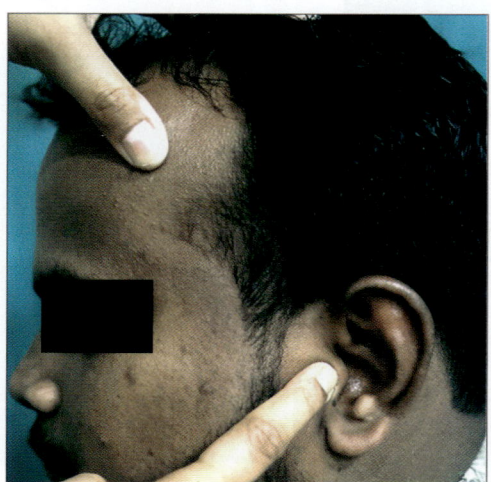

a. What is the test being performed here?
b. What is Hennebert's sign?
c. When is this test false negative?
d. In which condition do we get a negative result of the test.

Q11. Observe the image below:

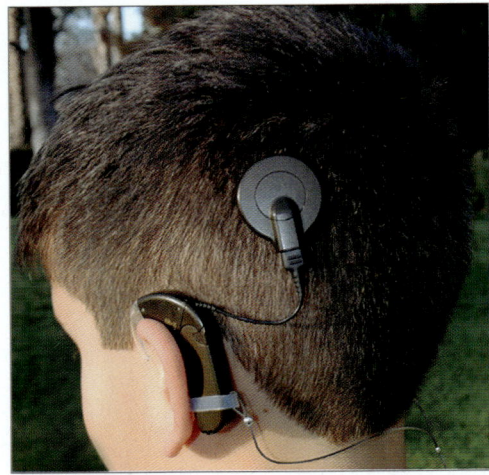

a. What is the device being worn by this patient known as?
b. Name two surgical techniques which can be done for placing this device.
c. Name one surgical complication of this procedure.

Q12. Observe the images given below:

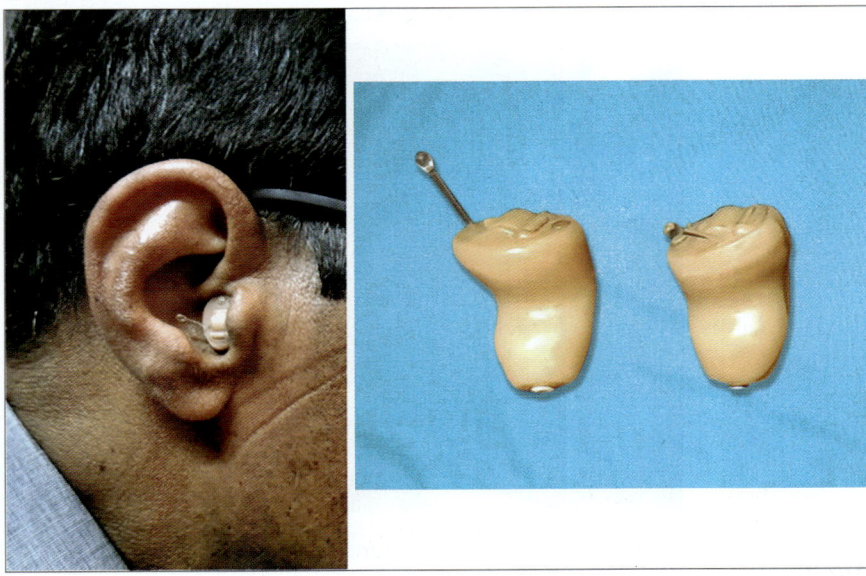

a. What is the device being worn by this patient?
b. What is the type of hearing loss this patient is having, for which he is using this device?

CHAPTER 3: Clinical Methods

ANSWERS

Ans 1:
  a. Bone conduction (BC) being checked
  b. Mastoid process (hair-free area)

Ans 2:
  a. The cotton wool should form a fluff in front, Jobson-Horne probe/stick extending only halfway into the cotton wool. Protrusion of the cotton-wool beyond the end of the Jobson-Horne probe/stick will ensure that if the mop touches either the deep canal skin or the tympanic membrane, no damage will occur or pain be felt
  b. Wait and watch. Traumatic perforations generally heal by themselves

Ans 3:
  a. Otoscopy
  b. Pinna is pulled postero-superiorly (upward, backward and laterally)
  c. Check for tragal tenderness, because if present, otoscopy will be painful for the patient. Hence, it should be done gently and cautiously

Ans 4:
  a. 'A': Tympanosclerotic patch
     'B': Middle ear mucosa
  b. Chronic otitis media with central perforation (mucosal type, inactive)
  c. Perforation in which there is a surrounding rim of pars tensa present all around

Ans 5:
  a. Acute suppurative otitis media (ASOM)—cartwheel sign
  b. *Streptococcus pneumoniae* (30%), *Haemophilus influenzae* (20%), *Moraxella catarrhalis* (12%)

Ans 6:
  a. Tubercular otitis media
  b. False (disease has painless ear discharge—earache is characteristically absent in cases of tubercular otitis media)
  c. Systemic antitubercular drugs are mandatory, along with local treatment

Ans 7:
  a. Syringing of the ear
  b. Patient may experience dizziness episode/vertigo after syringing

Ans 8:
  a. Left sided facial palsy
  b. Steroids
  c. Labyrinthine segment

Ans 9:
   a. Acute mastoiditis (ironed out appearance of the mastoid)
   b. Bruising over the mastoid/mastoid ecchymosis (in head trauma)
   c. Furunculosis of the external auditory canal

Ans 10:
   a. Fistula test
   b. Hennebert's sign: A false positive fistula test (i.e., positive fistula test without the presence of a fistula) is seen in congenital syphilis and in about 25% cases of Meniere's disease
   c. A false negative fistula test is seen when the cholesteatoma covers the site of fistula and does not allow pressure changes to be transmitted to the labyrinth
   d. Dead labyrinth

Ans 11:
   a. Cochlear implant (external parts of the cochlear implant being seen—the microphone with speech processor, the external magnet and transmitter)
   b. i. Posterior tympanotomy technique
      ii. Veria technique
   c. Wound infection, device failure, facial nerve injury, CSF fistula (may write any one)

Ans 12:
   a. Hearing aid (completely-in-canal type of hearing aid)
   b. Sensorineural hearing loss/mixed hearing loss

Surgical Procedures

Q1. The following image shows an initial step of a surgery being performed:

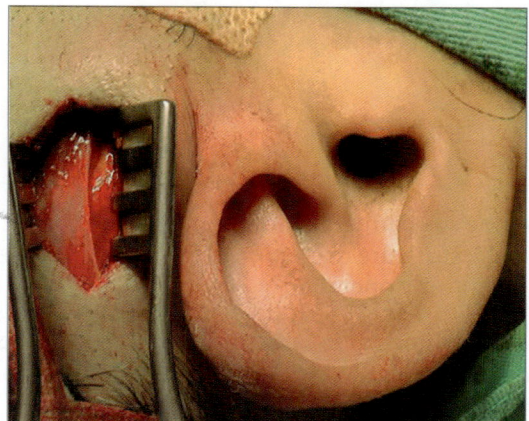

a. What is the graft being harvested in the picture above?
b. Name two surgeries it can be used in.
c. Mention three advantages of this graft.

Q2. The following Figures show incisions for ear surgery:

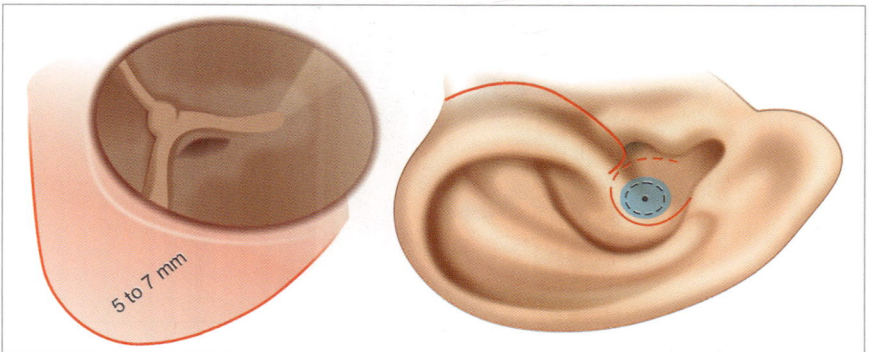

Figure 1   Figure 2

a. What are the two incisions shown in Figure 1 and Figure 2?
b. How many parts are there in the incision shown in Figure 2?
c. Where is Wilde's incision made?

Q3. The following image is showing the cavity after complete mastoidectomy:

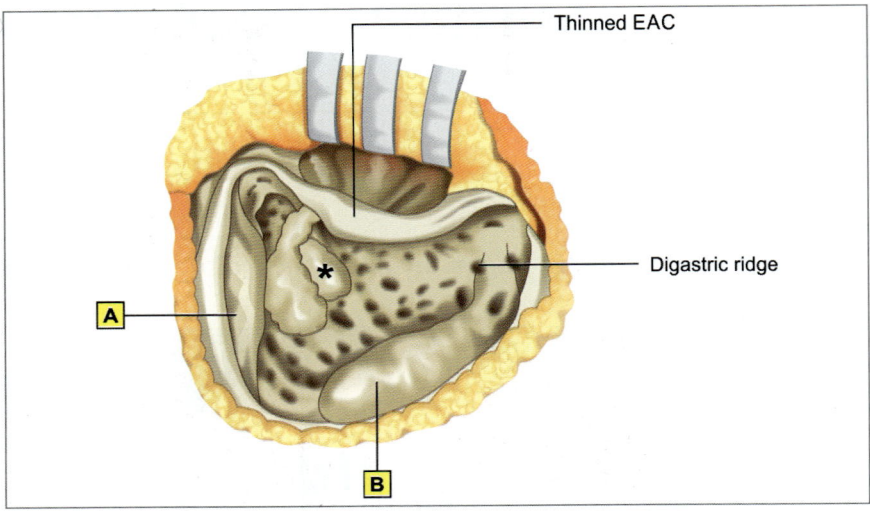

a. Answer the structures labelled 'A' and 'B'.
b. What is the structure marked '*' in the diagram?
c. What is Schwartz operation?

Q4. The following image is showing a step in the surgery for otosclerosis:

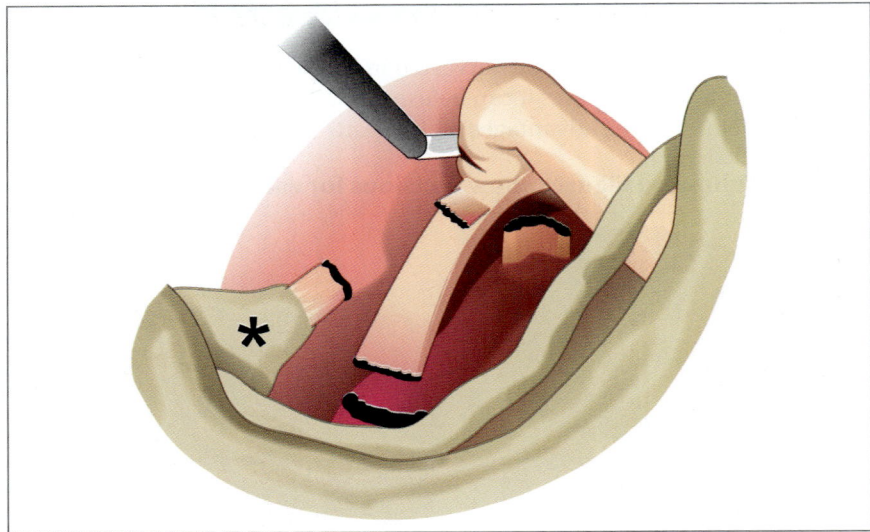

a. What is the surgery being performed?
b. What is the structure marked with '*' being shown in the image?
c. What is the step of the surgery that is being shown in the image?

Q5. The following picture shows the intervention done in a 13-year-old girl:

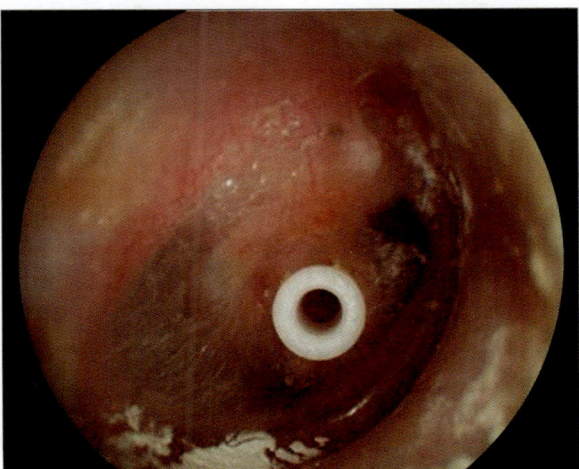

a. What is the white structure shown in the picture?
b. Name the condition of the ear in which it is used.
c. Which quadrant of the tympanic membrane is it placed in?

ANSWERS

Ans 1:
   a. Temporalis fascia graft
   b. (i) Tympanoplasty (ii) Intact canal wall mastoidectomy
   c. (i) Easy to harvest, (ii) Low BMR, (iii) Autologous material

Ans 2:
   a. Figure 1: Rosen's endomeatal incision
      Figure 2: Lempert's endaural incision
   b. 2 parts: i. In the canal, ii. In the incisura terminalis
   c. Postaural region (0.5 cm to 1 cm behind the post-aural groove)

Ans 3:
   a. 'A': Middle fossa tegmen
      'B': Sigmoid sinus
   b. '*': Lateral semi-circular canal
   c. Cortical mastoidectomy is also known as simple or complete mastoidectomy or Schwartz operation

Ans 4:
   a. Stapedotomy/Stapedectomy
   b. '*': Pyramidal process
   c. Step: Separation of the incudostapedial joint with a proprietary knife. Many surgeons prefer to separate the joint before incising the stapedial tendon in view of more stability during disarticulation. The intact stapedial tendon counteracts movements during the separation. Excessive lateral movement of the incus is avoided

Ans 5:
   a. Grommet
   b. OME (otitis media with effusion)
   c. Antero-inferior quadrant

Development

Q1. Regarding the development of the auricle, answer the following:

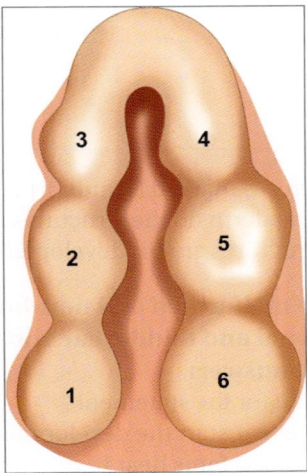

a. When does the development of the auricle start?
b. When does the auricle attain adult shape?
c. What are the six tubercles shown in the figure above known as?
d. What do parts numbered 3 and 6 give rise to?

Q2. The given figure shows the development of the external and middle ear.

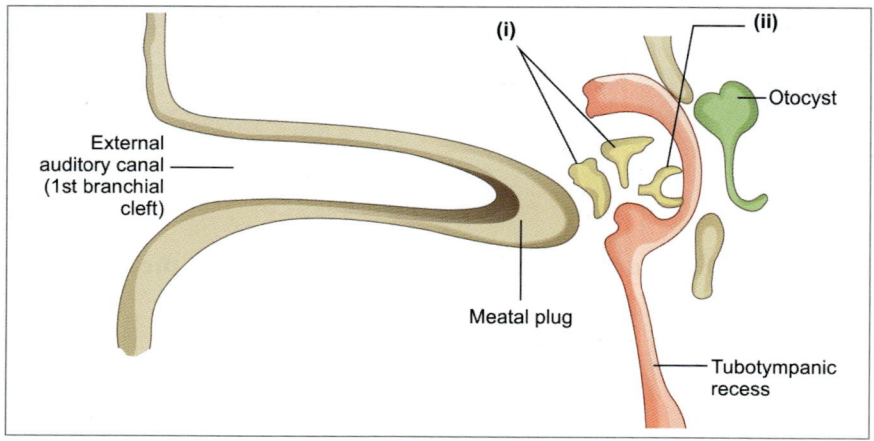

a. Label the structures marked (i) and (ii)
b. Which arch mesoderm do the structures labelled (i) come from?
c. From which structures are (ii) developed?

Q3. Inner ear may be malformed and non-functional in the presence of a normal external and middle ear and vice versa. With regards to this statement, answer:
a. Brief explanation for the statement.
b. When does inner ear start the development?
c. By what time can the fetus hear in the womb of the mother?

Q4. With regards to the development of the mastoid, answer:

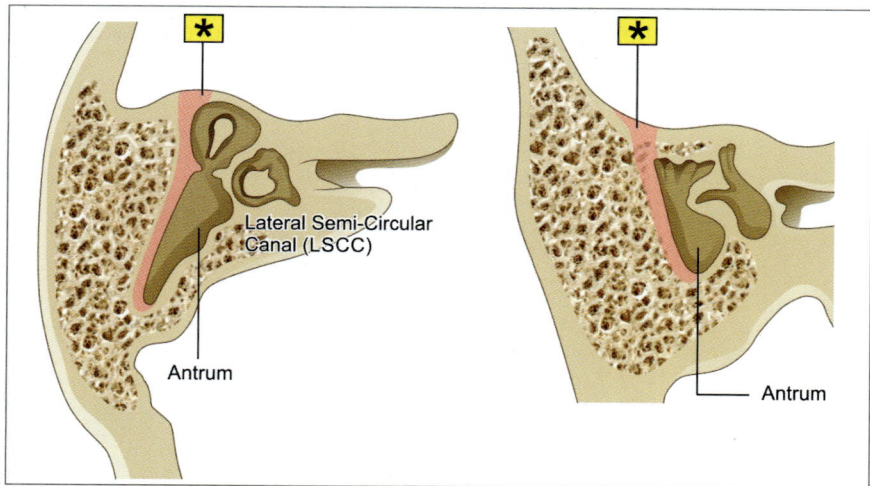

a. Label the structure marked with "*" in the diagram above.
b. Name one area of the temporal bone, which can be accessed by the translabyrinthine approach.

CHAPTER 5: Development

Q5. The following is the image of a 3-year-old boy with history of recurrent infections:

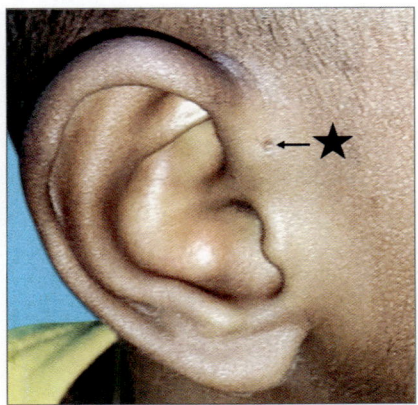

a. What is the condition being shown in the picture above marked with the star?
b. What is the etiology?
c. What is the treatment of choice?

Q6. The following photographs are of a 1-year-old boy presenting to the ENT OPD:

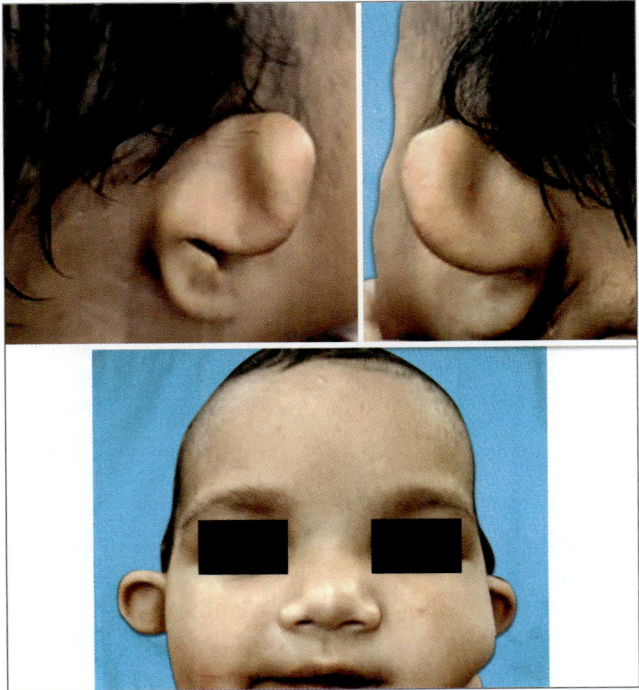

a. What is deformity of the external ear known as?
b. Why does it occur?

Q7. A 7-year-old boy came with the complaint of poor speech development. On examination, the following was found:

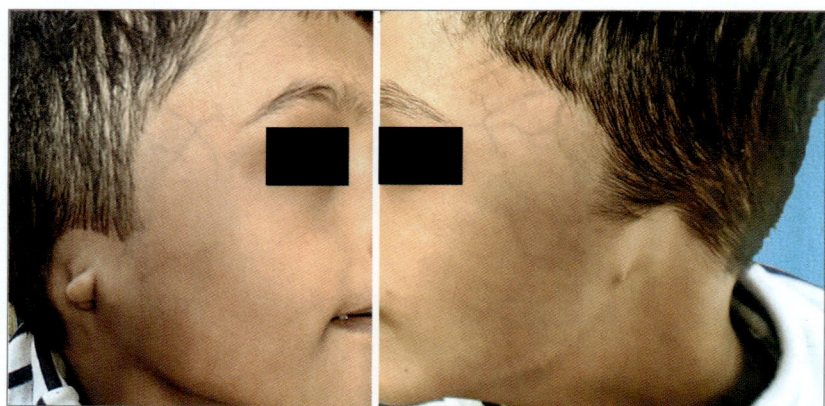

Figure A   Figure B

    a. What is the diagnosis of the Figure 'A'?
    b. What is being shown in Figure 'B'?
    c. What is the investigation that should be ordered to this boy?

Q8. Observe the images below relating to the embryogenesis of the inner ear:

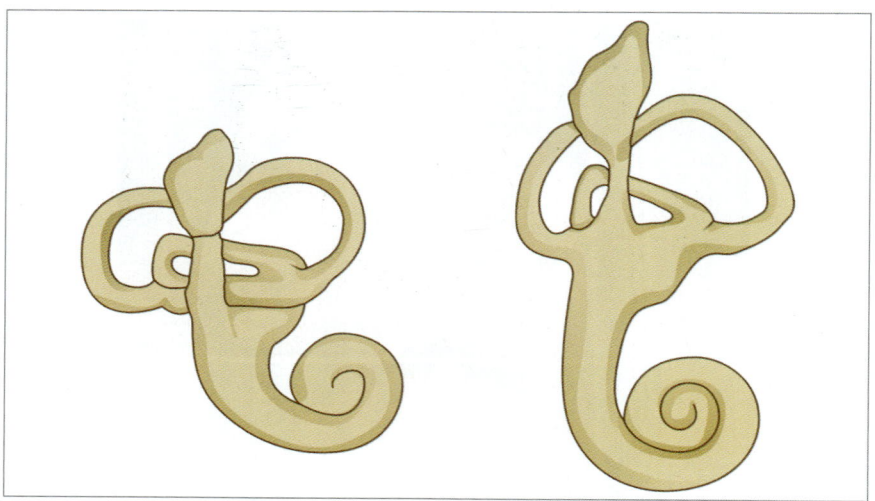

Figure A   Figure B

    a. The Figure 'B' shows the developmental stage at 8 weeks. What is it showing?
    b. What classical finding is shown in Figure 'A'?
    c. Mention one symptom that can be present in a child with the inner ear shown in 'A'.

CHAPTER 5: Development

ANSWERS

Ans 1:
- a. 6 weeks of gestational life
- b. 20 weeks
- c. Hillocks of His
- d. Part 3–Helix, Part 6–Lobule

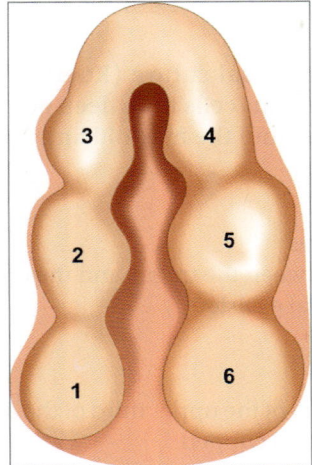

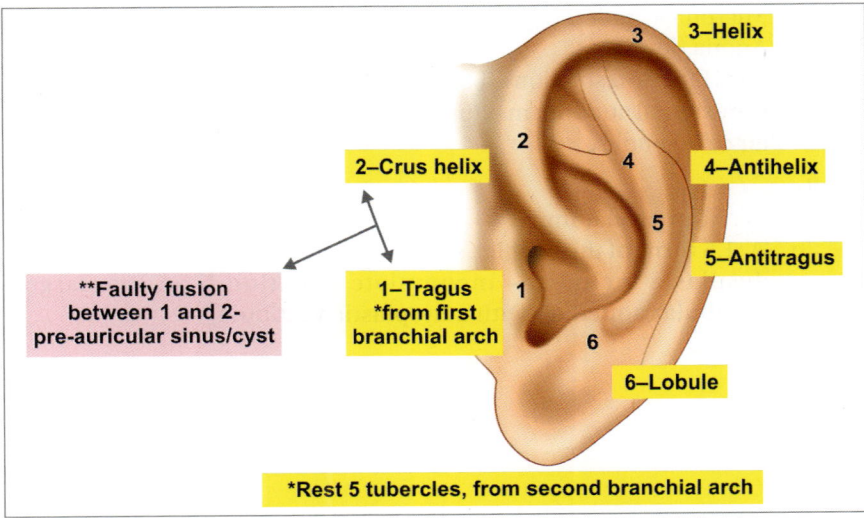

Ans 2:
- a. (i) Malleus, incus; (ii) Stapes
- b. Mesoderm of first branchial arch
- c. Stapes superstructure–second arch derivative; stapes footplate and annular ligament–otic capsule

SECTION 1: Ear

Ans 3:
- a. The inner ear develops independently of the external and middle ears. **Ectoderm** in hindbrain thickens—**Auditory placode** formed–Invagination–**Auditory vesicle or otocyst** forms–differentiate into endolymphatic duct, sac; utricle and semicircular canals (pars superior); saccule and cochlea (pars inferior)
- b. 3rd week
- c. 20 weeks (as cochlea develops by then)

Ans 4:
- a. "*" – Petro-squamosal suture (Koerner's septum): Separating superficial squamous cells from deep petrosal cells. It needs to be removed to enter into the mastoid antrum
- b. Petrous apex

Ans 5:
- a. Preauricular sinus
- b. Faulty fusion between the tragus and the crus helix
- c. Complete surgical excision

Ans 6:
- a. Lop ear
- b. Due to hypoplasia of the upper third of the auricle – upper portion of the pinna or helix is cupped

Ans 7:
- a. Microtia – grade 3 (right side)
- b. Anotia (left side)
- c. HRCT (high-resolution CT scan) of temporal bone: To see the status of the external auditory meatus, middle ear, ossicles, inner ear, mastoid air cell complex

Ans 8:
- a. 'B': Normal anatomy
- b. 'A': 1.5 turns of the cochlea seen in Mondini's dysplasia (Mondini's dysplasia includes – Incomplete partition II with enlarged vestibular aqueduct with a dysplastic vestibule)

CHAPTER 6
Audio-Vestibulometry

Q1. Answer the following with respect to tuning forks.

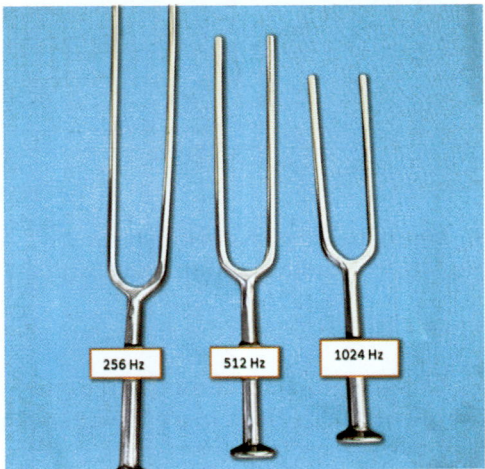

a. Name one frequency of the tuning fork from the above figure which is considered ideal for routine clinical practice.
b. Why is that frequency considered ideal?
c. What is the distance from the opening of the external auditory canal that the tuning forks are placed at while testing?

Q2. Name the clinical condition/type of hearing loss, in which we get each of the following findings on tuning fork tests:
a. A false negative Rinne's test?
b. Lengthened Schwabach's test?
c. Negative Bing test?
d. Positive Gelle's test?

Q3. The following image shows an audiogram done on a 33-year-old lady:

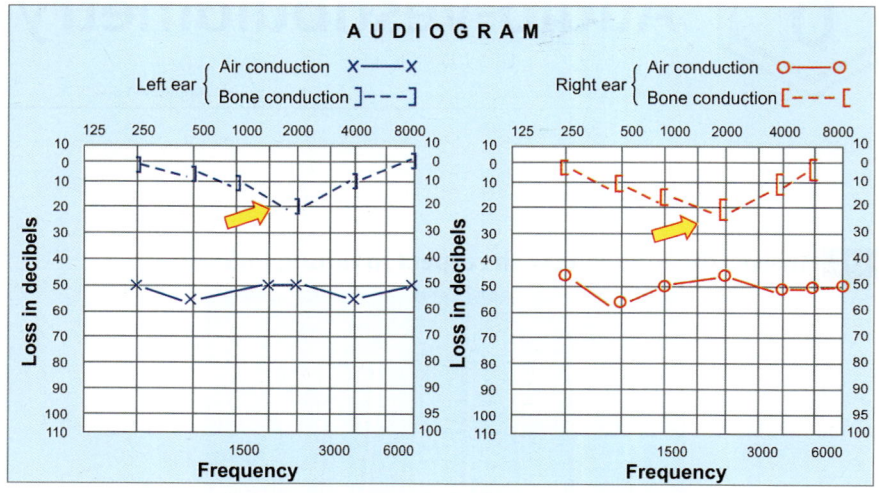

a. What is the type of hearing loss being shown?
b. What is the classical finding being marked with the arrow in the left ear?
c. Give 2 probable diagnosis from the audiogram above.

Q4. The following image shows an audiogram done on a 53-year-old gentleman who works as a clerk in a railway station:

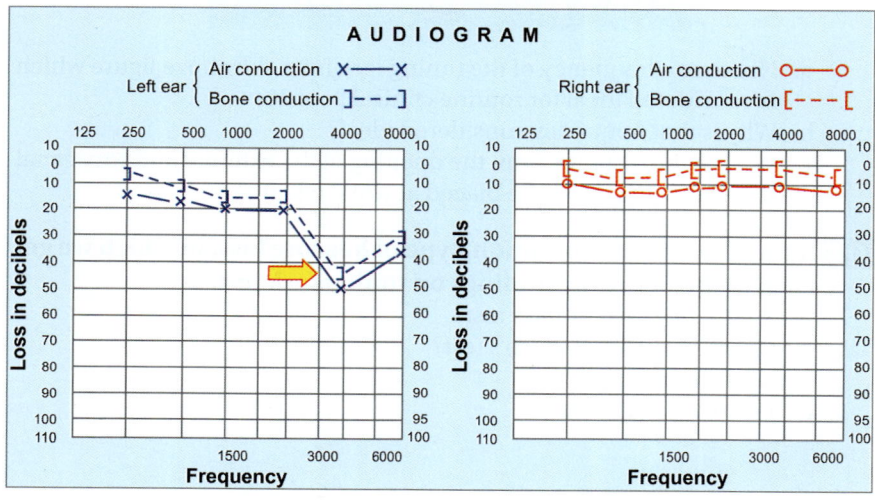

a. What is being shown by the arrow marked in the audiogram of left ear?
b. What is the diagnosis of the left side?
c. What is the diagnosis of the right ear?

Q5. The following image shows an audiogram done on a 70-year-old gentleman who has come to the OPD with the complaint of hearing loss:

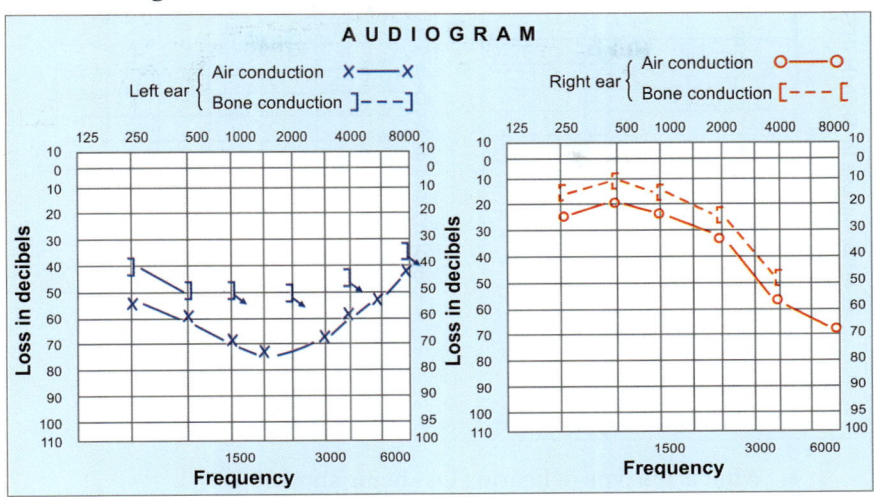

a. What is the type of hearing loss in the right ear?
b. What is the diagnosis of the right side?
c. What treatment advice will you give to the patient?
d. What is the diagnosis of the left side?

Q6. The following image shows a tympanogram in a 12-year-old girl with complaint of reduced hearing:

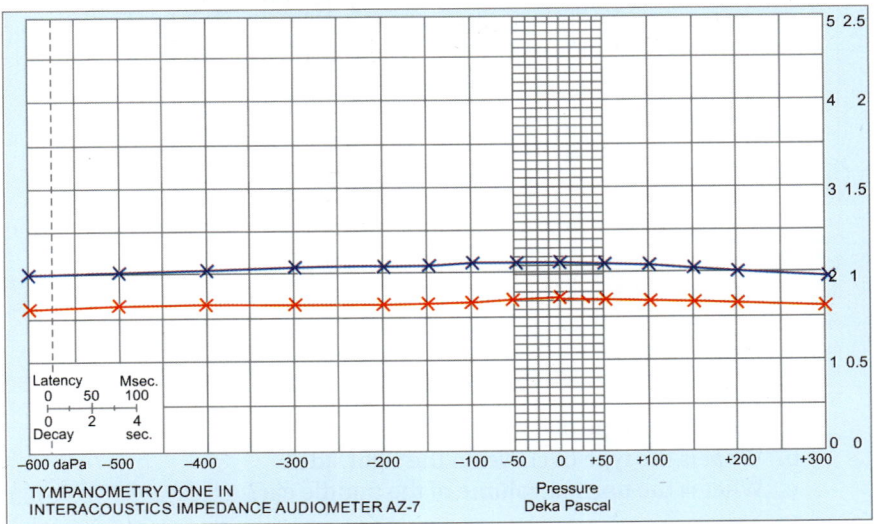

a. What is the type of audiogram curve being shown in the image above?
b. Name two conditions in which this type of curve is seen.

Q7. The following shows an audiogram:

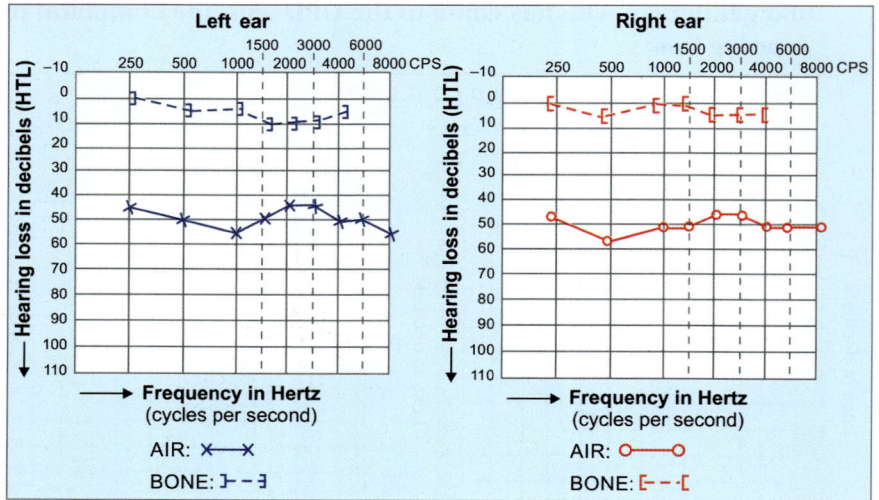

a. What is the type of hearing loss being shown?
b. Give 2 disease conditions in which this type of audiogram can be seen.

Q8. The following image shows a tympanogram:

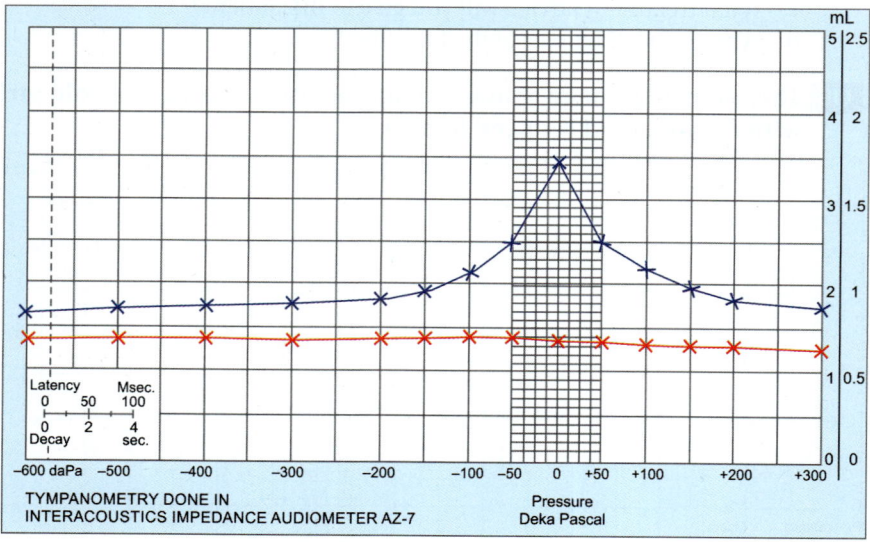

a. What is the type of curve on the left side?
b. What is the type of curve on the right side?
c. What is the normal volume of the middle ear?

Q9. The following is an audiogram of a 20-year-old boy with complaints of tinnitus and itching sensation in both ears following an episode of upper respiratory tract infection:

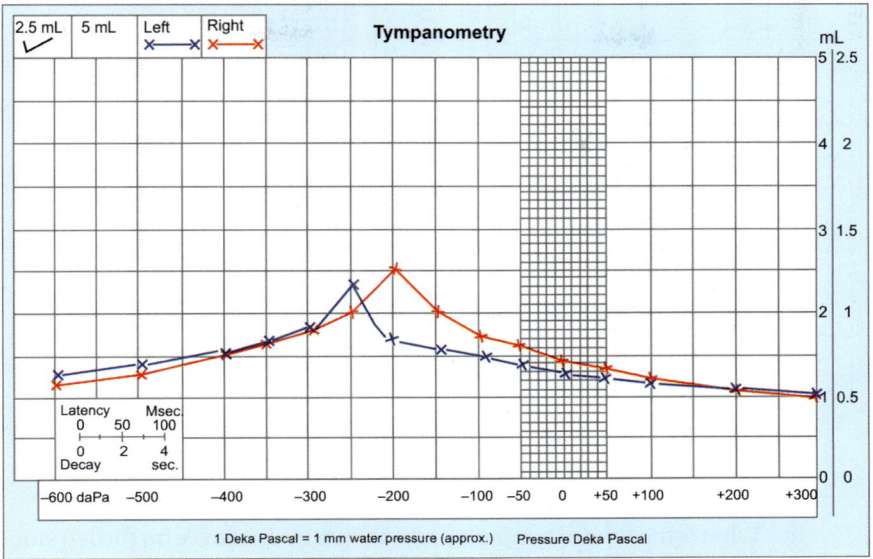

a. What is the type of curve on the left and right side each?
b. What is the possible cause of this type of curve?

Q10. The following is an audiogram:

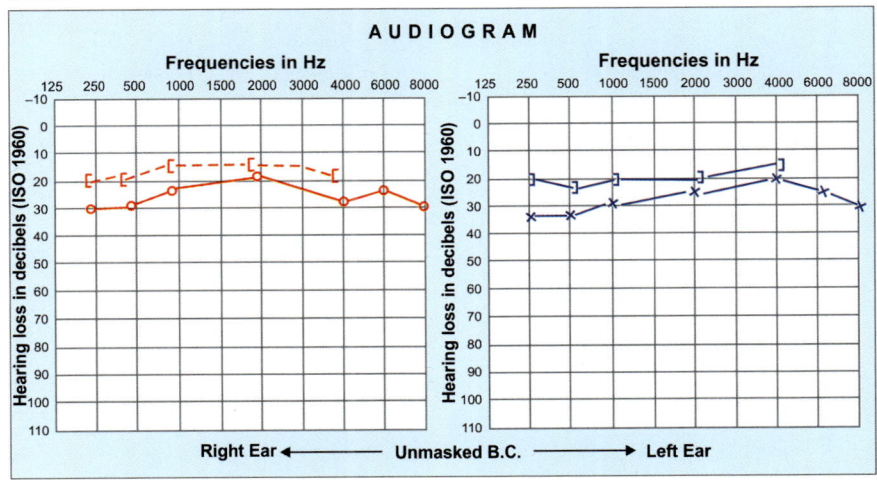

a. What is the diagnosis from the curves shown?
b. While testing the right ear for assessment of the hearing threshold, masking is performed on which side—right ear/left ear?
c. What is the type of audiogram seen in early Meniere's disease?

Q11. The following image shows a tympanogram:

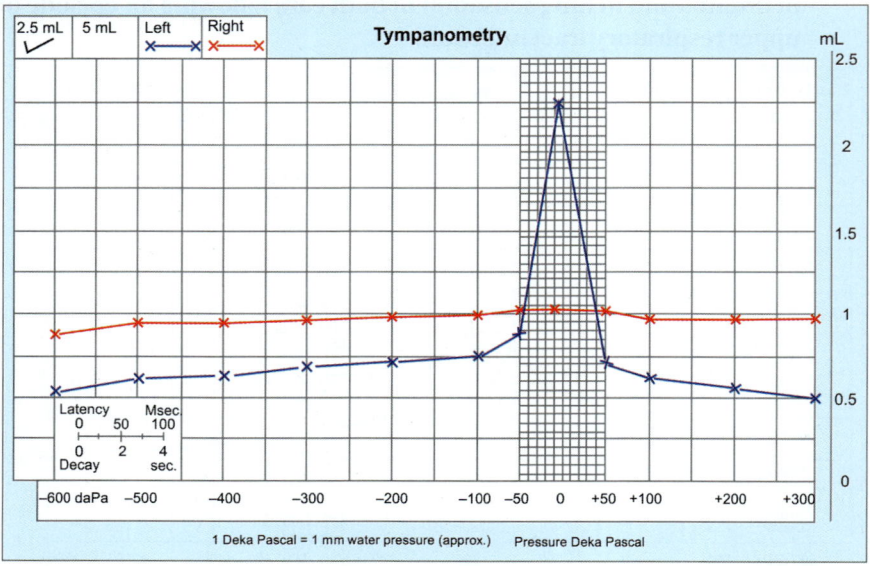

a. What is the type of tympanogram shown in this curve on the left side?
b. What could be the possible explanation of this curve?
c. What is the tympanogram curve seen in otosclerosis?

Q12. The following image shows a chart after a test was done in a patient with complaints of vertigo:

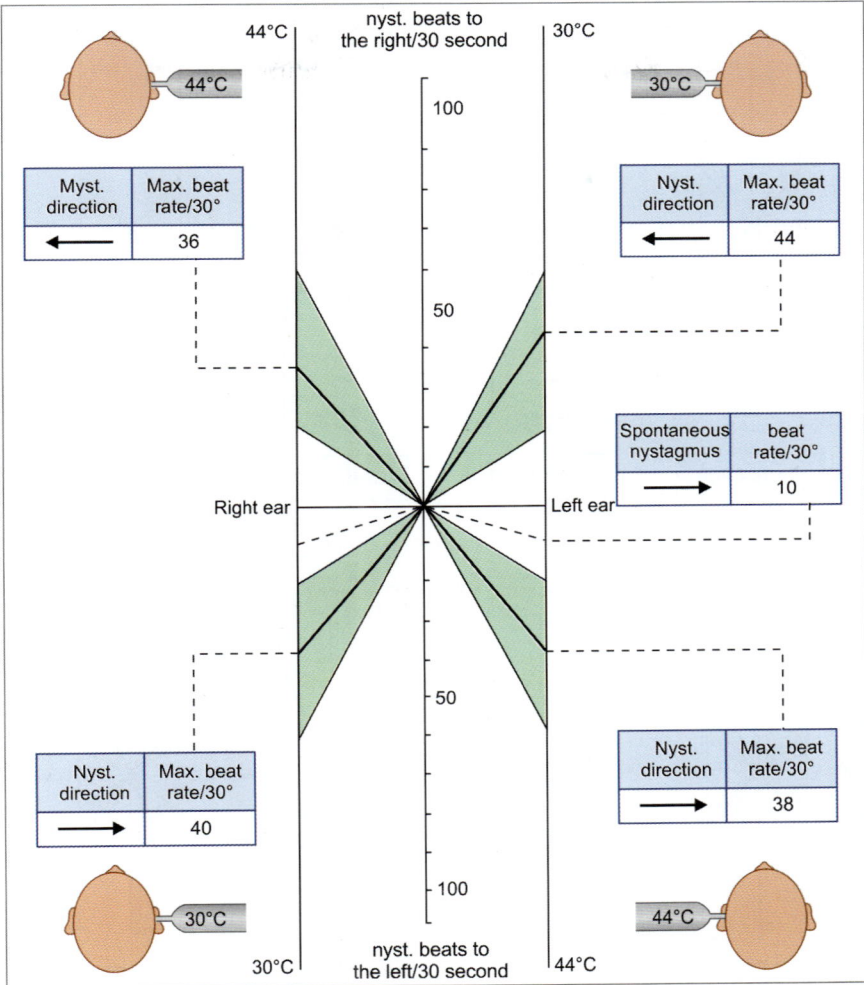

a. What is this chart known as?
b. What is the test performed on the patient for which this chart is made?
c. What is the coding used in this chart for indicating the activity of the vestibular system?

Q13. The following image shows the various coding:

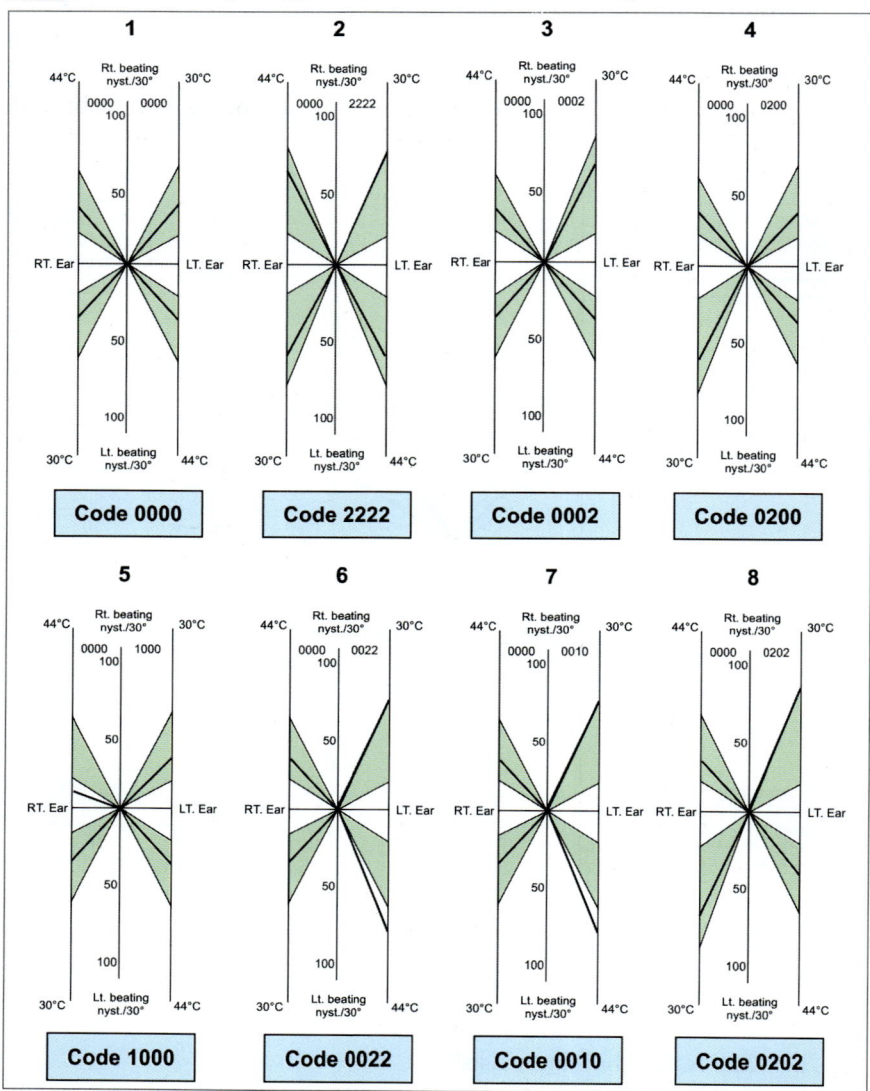

a. What is the interpretation of the code 0000?
b. What is the interpretation of the code 0011?

ANSWERS

Ans 1:
a. 512 Hz
b. Tuning forks of lower frequency produce a sense of bone vibration while those of higher frequencies have a shorter decay time and are thus not routinely preferred
c. 2 cm

Ans 2:
a. Severe unilateral sensorineural hearing loss
b. Conductive hearing loss
c. Conductive hearing loss (e.g., otosclerosis). Bing's test is positive in normal or sensorineural hearing loss
d. Normal or sensorineural hearing loss. Gelle's test is negative in conductive hearing loss (e.g., ossicular chain fixation or discontinuity)

> **REMEMBER: BING & GELLE'S TEST…GO HAND IN HAND!**
> "NEGATIVE" IN CONDUCTIVE HEARING LOSS.
> "POSITIVE" IN NORMAL OR SENSORINEURAL HEARING LOSS.

Ans 3:
a. Conductive hearing loss
b. Carhart's notch: Dip in BC at 2000Hz
c. Otosclerosis, malleus head ankylosis

Ans 4:
a. Dip in BC at 4000Hz
b. Noise-induced hearing loss
c. Normal hearing

Ans 5:
a. High frequency sensorineural hearing loss
b. Presbycusis
c. Hearing aid trial
d. Congenital deafness: Trough shaped audiogram

Ans 6:
a. 'B' type tympanogram curve
b. (i) Tympanic membrane perforation (chronic otitis media)
   (ii) Glue ear

Ans 7:
a. Bilateral moderate conductive hearing loss
b. (i) Chronic otitis media
   (ii) Tympanosclerosis

Ans 8:
- a. Left side: Normal 'A' type curve
- b. Right side: 'B' type curve (flat)
- c. It is considered abnormal when volume larger than 2.0 ml in children, or 2.5 ml in adults

Ans 9:
- a. Left side: 'C' type curve
  Right side: 'C' type curve
- b. It is suggestive of Eustachian tube dysfunction

Ans 10:
- a. Normal hearing (both sides)
- b. Left ear is to be masked while testing the right ear
- c. Rising audiogram

Ans 11:
- a. A_d type of audiogram: left
- b. It is suggestive of ossicular chain discontinuity
- c. As type of audiogram in otosclerosis

Ans 12:
- a. Butterfly chart/Butterfly vestibulometry: method of simple and quantitative representation of the results of the bi-thermal caloric test
- b. Fitzgerald-Hallpike bithermal caloric test
- c. 0: Normal caloric response, 1: Hypoactive, 2: Hyperactive

Ans 13:
- a. Code 0000: Normal caloric responses on right and left
- b. Code 0011: Both normal caloric responses on right ear, both hypoactive responses on left ear

NOSE AND PARANASAL SINUSES

SECTION 2

SECTION OUTLINE

7. Anatomy
8. Physiology
9. Clinical Methods
10. Surgical Procedures
11. Development

Anatomy

Q1. The following diagram shows the anatomy of the external nose:

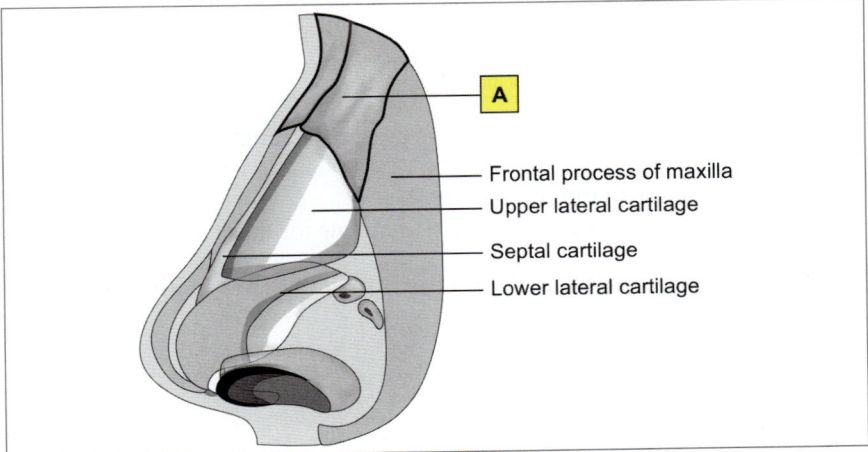

a. What is the structure being asked in the diagram above?
b. What are the boundaries of the internal nasal valve?

SECTION 2: Nose and Paranasal Sinuses

Q2. The following image shows the structures on the lateral wall of the nose:

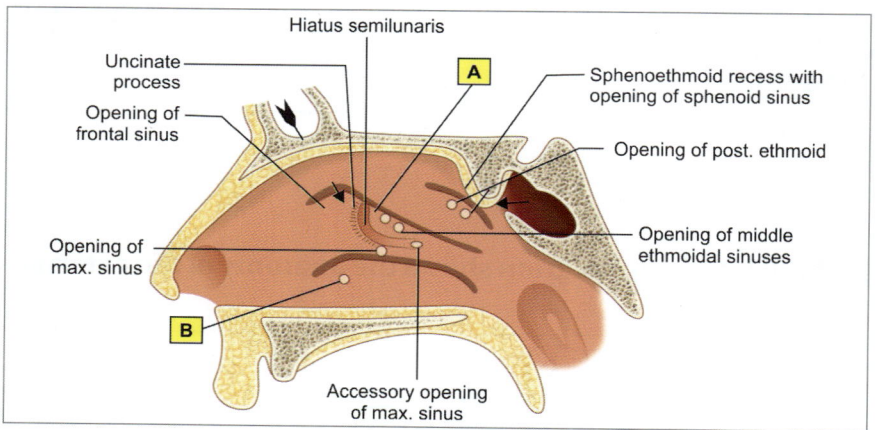

a. The structure labelled 'A' shows the largest anterior ethmoid air cell. What is it?
b. Name the structure marked as 'B'.
c. What are the 3 major nerves responsible for nasal sensation?

Q3. The following diagram shows the different types of attachment of the uncinate process:

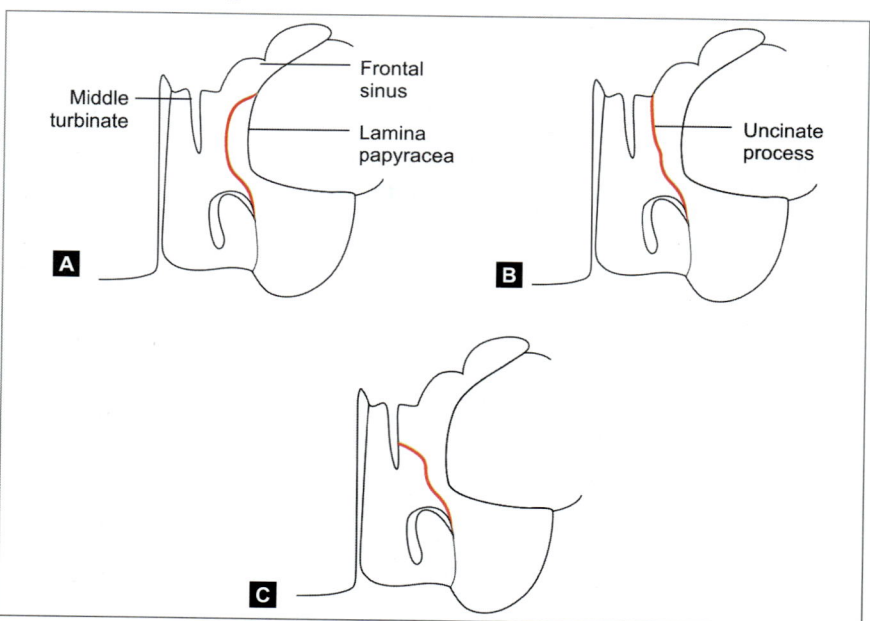

a. Which among the three types shown is the most common type of attachment?
b. Lateral and posterior pneumatization of a posterior ethmoid cell, gives rise to a cell overlying the optic nerve. What is this cell called?

CHAPTER 7: Anatomy

Q4. The following illustration is of a coronal section through the middle meatus:

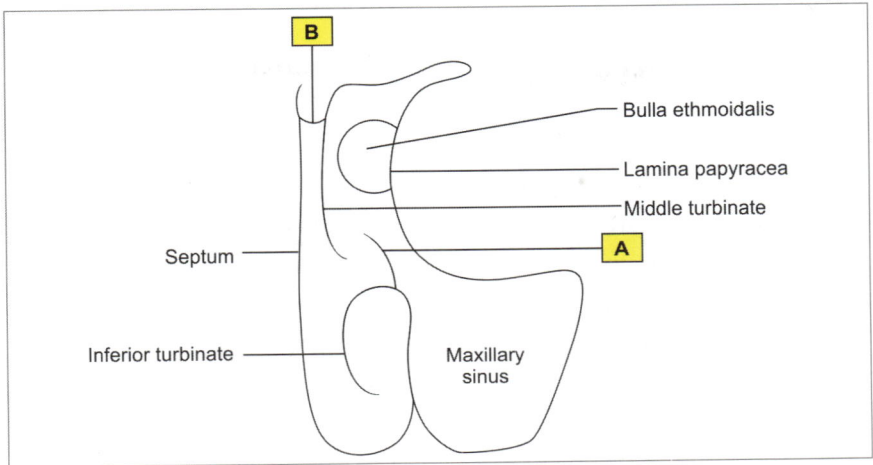

a. What are the structures marked as 'A' and 'B'?
b. Answer the following with respect to the middle turbinate:

Part of middle turbinate	Plane of orientation	Attachment
Anterior one-third	Sagittal plane	(i)
Middle one-third	(ii)	(iii)
Posterior one-third	(iv)	Lateral nasal wall

Q5. The following is a CT scan of nose and PNS of a 22-year-old lady:

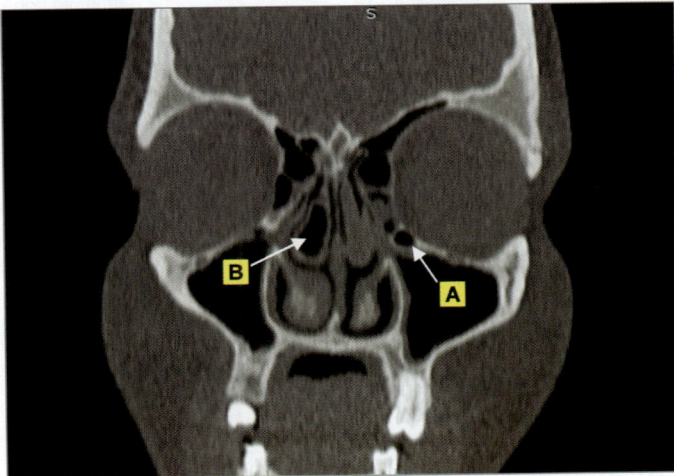

a. What is the structure marked by 'A'?
b. What is the anatomical variant of the middle turbinate being shown by 'B' known as?
c. What is a paradoxically bent middle turbinate?

Q6. The following shows the blood supply of the nasal septum:

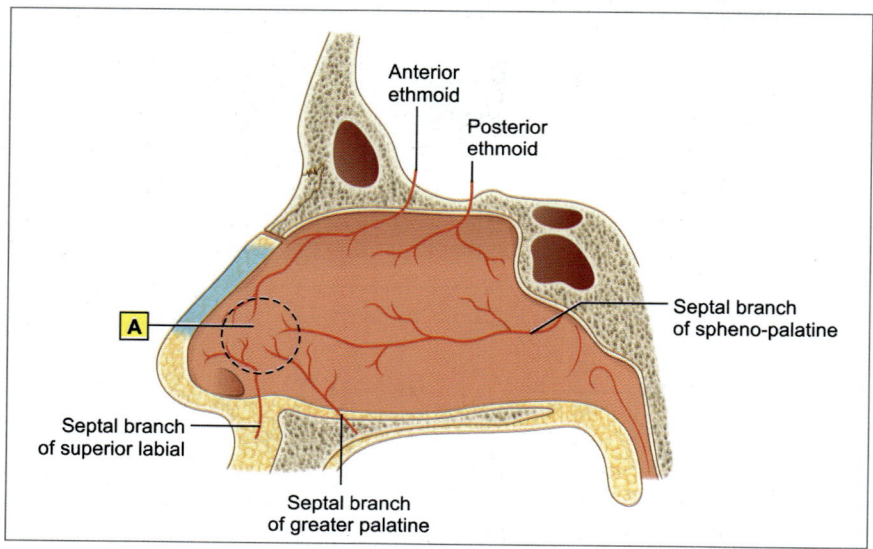

a. What does 'A' depict?
b. What is Woodruff's plexus. Where is it located?
c. What does TESPAL stand for?
d. Hypertension generally causes anterior epistaxis. True/False?

Q7. The following image shows the anatomy of the nasal septum:

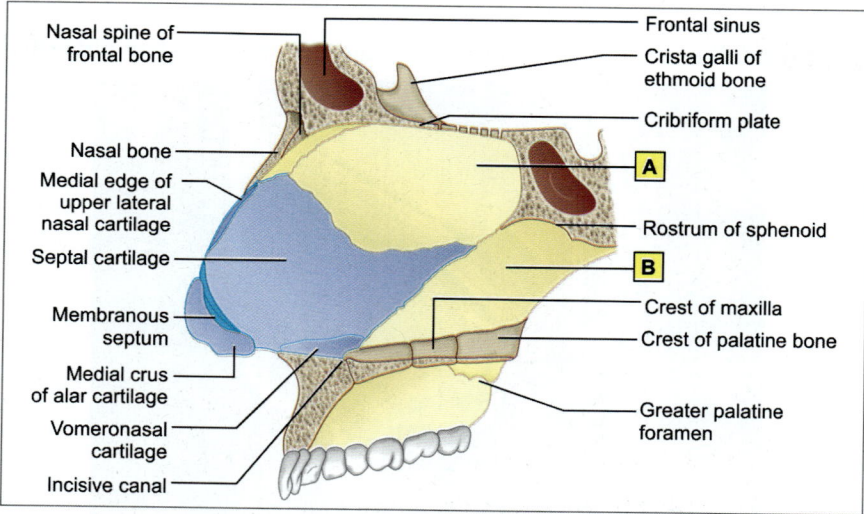

a. What are the 3 parts of the nasal septum?
b. What are the structures being shown by 'A' and 'B'?
c. What is septal swell body?

Q8. The following is an image of a patient who came with an inflammation of the vestibule:

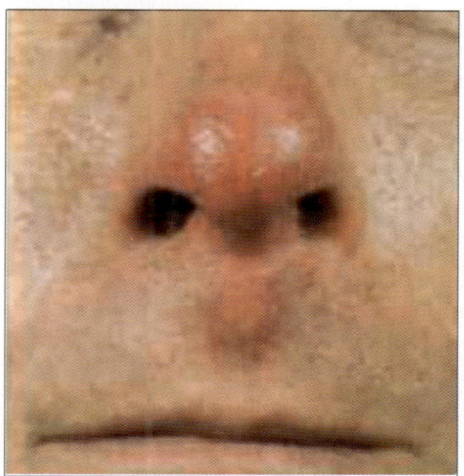

a. What is this condition called?
b. What is this area known as?
c. Why is it called so?

ANSWERS

Ans 1:
   a. Nasal bones
   b. Internal nasal valve: Laterally—lower border of upper lateral cartilage and fibrofatty tissue and anterior border of the inferior turbinate
   Medially—cartilaginous septum
   Caudally—floor of pyriform aperture

Ans 2:
   a. 'A': Bulla ethmoidalis
   b. 'B': Opening of the nasolacrimal duct
   c. Nerve supply:
      i. Anterior ethmoidal nerve
      ii. Branches of infraorbital nerve
      iii. Branches of sphenopalatine ganglion

Ans 3:
   a. A: Attachment of uncinate process to the medial wall of the orbit (85%)—leading to a frontal recess drainage pathway medial to the uncinate
   b. Onodi cell

Ans 4:
   a. 'A': Uncinate process
      'B': Cribriform plate
   b. (i) Skull base (at the lateral lamella)
      (ii) Coronal plane
      (iii) Lamina papyracea
      (iv) Axial plane

Anatomy of the middle turbinate:

Part of middle turbinate	Plane of orientation	Attachment
Anterior one-third	Sagittal plane	(I) **Skull base** (at lateral lamella - lateral edge of cribriform plate)
Middle one-third	(II) **Coronal plane**	(III) **Lamina papyraceae** (forms ground lamella separating anterior and posterior ethmoid air cells)
Posterior one-third	(IV) **Axial plane**	Lateral nasal wall

Ans 5:
   a. 'A': Haller cell
   b. 'B' Concha bullosa: pneumatized and ballooned up middle turbinate
   c. A middle turbinate having a sharp bend laterally instead of its usual smooth medial curvature is called paradoxically bent middle turbinate

Ans 6:
　　a. A: Little's area – Kisselbach's plexus
　　b. Plexus of veins. Situated inferior to the posterior end of the inferior turbinate
　　c. TESPAL—Transnasal endoscopic sphenopalatine artery ligation
　　d. False (hypertension generally causes posterior epistaxis)

Ans 7:
　　a. 3 parts: (i) Columellar septum, (ii) Membranous septum, (iii) Septum proper
　　b. 'A': Perpendicular plate of ethmoid
　　　 'B': Vomer
　　c. **Septal swell body:** Nasal septal swell body is a widened region of the anterior nasal septum, located anterior to the middle turbinate at the internal nasal valve (having increased amount of venous sinusoids)

Ans 8:
　　a. Nasal vestibulitis
　　b. Dangerous area of the face
　　c. Infections may be transmitted in a retrograde fashion through a valveless venous system to the cavernous sinus leading to cavernous sinus thrombosis (cranial nerves III, IV, V-1 and VI affected, leading to facial and periorbital edema, ptosis, proptosis, chemosis, discomfort and pain with eye muscle movement, papilledema, and loss of vision, diplopia, paresthesia around eyes, nose, forehead, loss of corneal reflex)

Physiology

Q1. The following diagram shows the mechanism of mucociliary clearance of the sinuses:

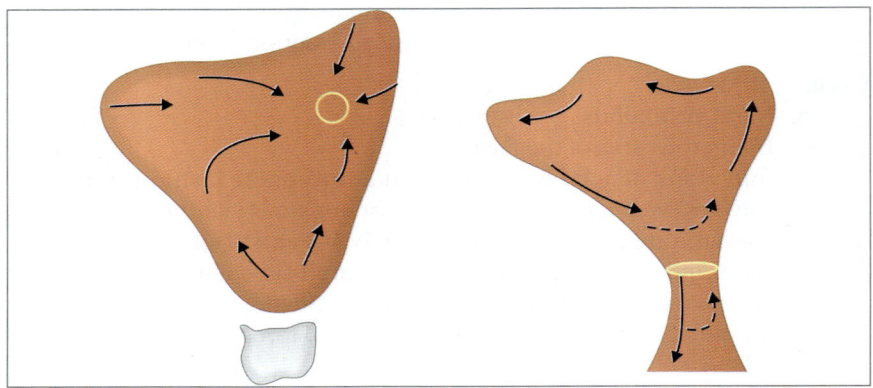

Figure A   Figure B

a. Figure A is depicting the mucociliary clearance of which sinus?
b. "Caldwell-Luc operation provides ventilation to the sinus shown in Figure A, but does not help in mucociliary clearance"—True/False?
c. Figure B is depicting the mucociliary clearance of which sinus? (**HINT!** Mention the side of the sinus too)
d. Where does mucus from the sphenoid sinus drain?

CHAPTER 8: Physiology

Q2. The following diagram shows the physiology of the nasal airflow:

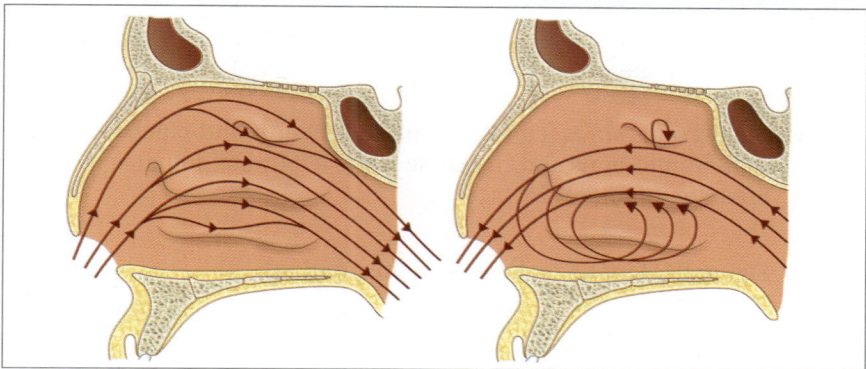

Figure A　　　　　　　　　　　　Figure B

a. Which is the airflow pattern during expiration?
b. "The nasal mucosa undergoes an alternating phase of congestion and decongestion, cyclically every 4–12 hours due to changes in the vascular activity in the venous sinusoids." What is this physiological activity known as?
c. Give one cause each of:
　(i) Rhinolalia clausa
　(ii) Rhinolalia aperta

Q3. Observe the photo below:

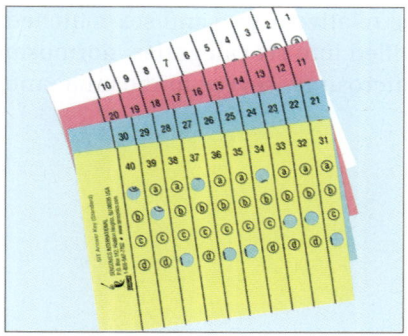

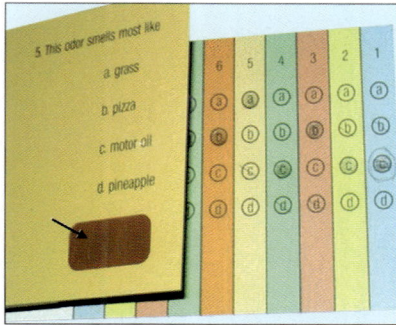

a. What is the booklet being shown in the images known as?
b. What is this used for?

ANSWERS

Ans 1:
   a. Maxillary sinus
   b. True
   c. Right frontal sinus (circulation of the mucus is anti-clockwise in the right frontal sinus and clockwise in the left frontal sinus)
   d. Sphenoethmoidal recess

Ans 2:
   a. Figure B (Figure A is showing for inspiration)
   b. Nasal cycle
   c. (i) Adenoid hypertrophy
      (ii) Submucous cleft palate

Ans 3:
   a. University of Pennsylvania Smell Identification Test (UPSIT), commercially known as Smell Identification Test
   b. To test olfaction
      The 40-item UPSIT is the most widely used olfactory test, having been administered to more than one million patients worldwide. It can be self-administered in 10–15 minutes by most patients, while in the waiting room. It can be scored by trained non-medical staff in less than a minute. It contains 4 booklets with 10 microencapsulated ('scratch and sniff') odorants in each (see the image in question). Test results are given in terms of a percentile score of a patient's performance relative to age and sex-matched controls. Olfaction can be classified into six categories: normosmia, mild microsmia, moderate microsmia, severe microsmia, anosmia and probable malingering

Clinical Methods

Q1. The image below shows a procedure being performed:

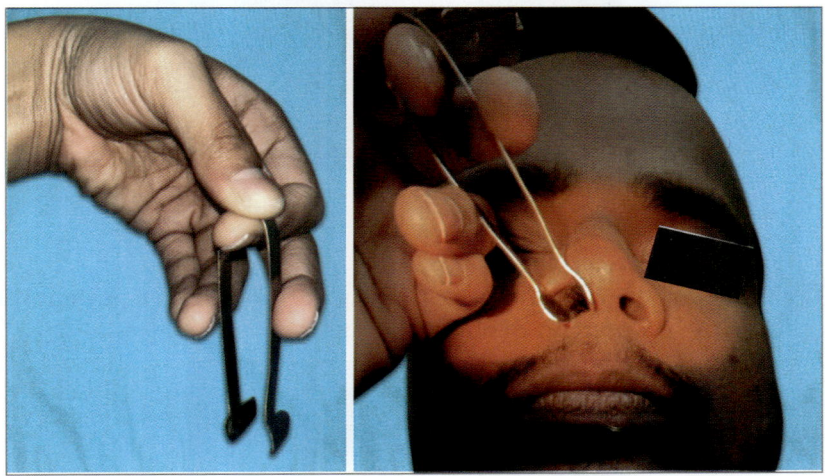

a. What is the test being performed here?
b. Draw and label the structures as seen in this test?
c. What is the instrument being used for this?

Q2. The image below shows a test being performed on a patient:

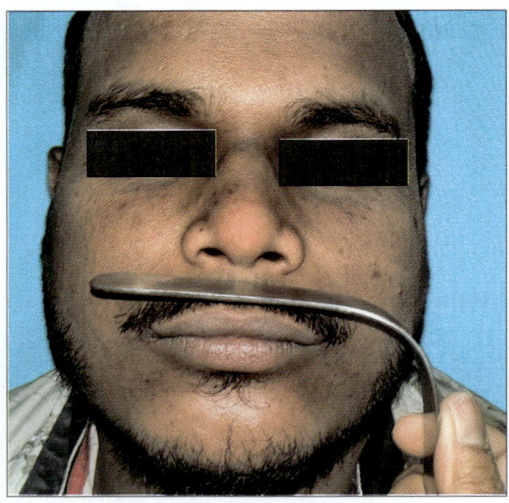

a. What is the test being shown?
b. How is this test interpreted?

Q3. The image below shows a test being performed on a patient with the complaint of nasal obstruction:

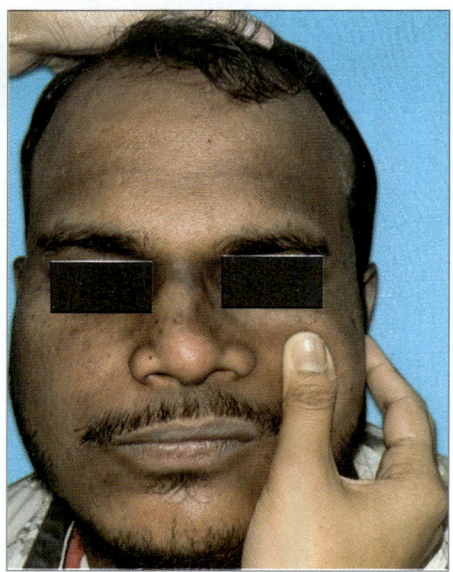

a. What is the test being shown?
b. "Improvement in the nasal airway, suggests the test is positive"—True/False?
c. This test checks which anatomical area of the nose?

Q4. The image below shows a test being performed on a patient:

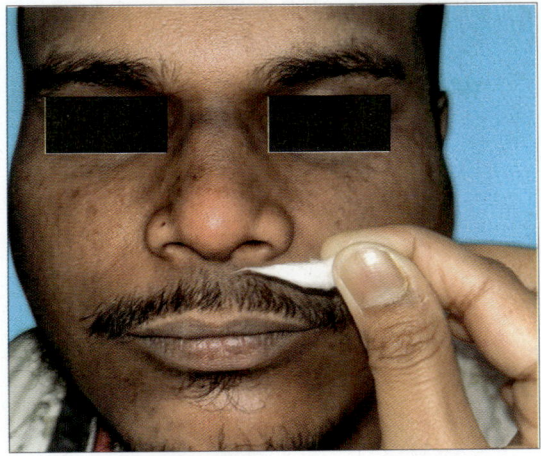

   a. What is the test being shown?
   b. How is this test interpreted?

Q5. The following images show some tests being performed on a patient:

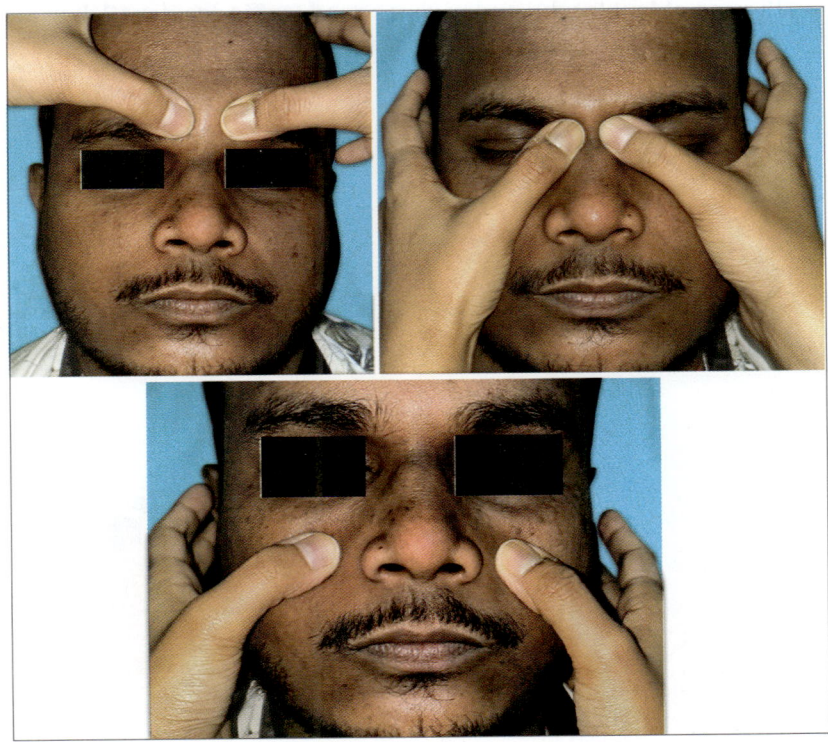

   a. What is being checked in these images?
   b. What is a positive finding in this test suggestive of?

SECTION 2: Nose and Paranasal Sinuses

Q6. The image below shows a test being performed in a patient:

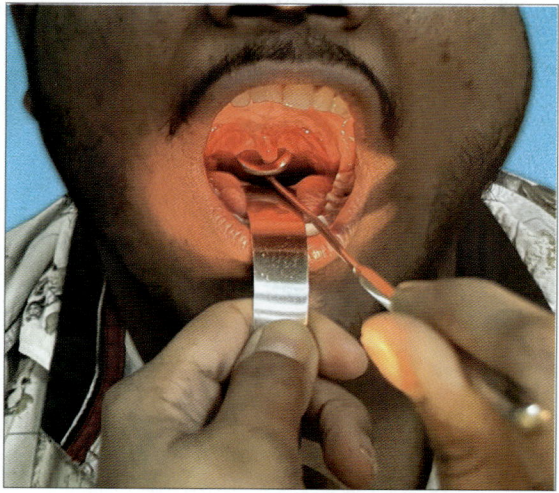

a. What is the test being performed here?
b. Draw and label the structures as seen in this test?

Q7. The following images show a technique being performed in a 25-year-old male who underwent a road traffic accident 7 days ago:

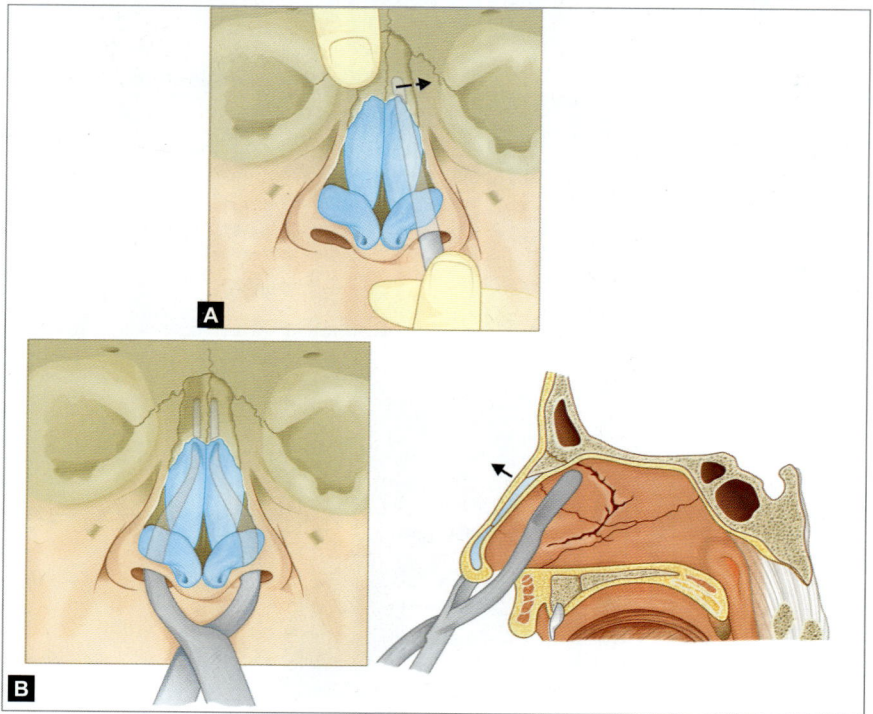

a. What is the procedure being shown in Figure 'A' and Figure 'B'?
b. What is the instrument being used in the Figure 'B'?
c. What is the best time to reduce a nasal fracture?

CHAPTER 9: Clinical Methods

Q8. The following image shows a 15-year-old boy with fullness on the right side of face and right side nasal obstruction. On palpation there is a diffuse, firm swelling on the right side of face.
   a. Give the two most probable diagnoses for this patient.
   b. What is the investigation you will order for the patient?
   c. From what does ameloblastoma arise?

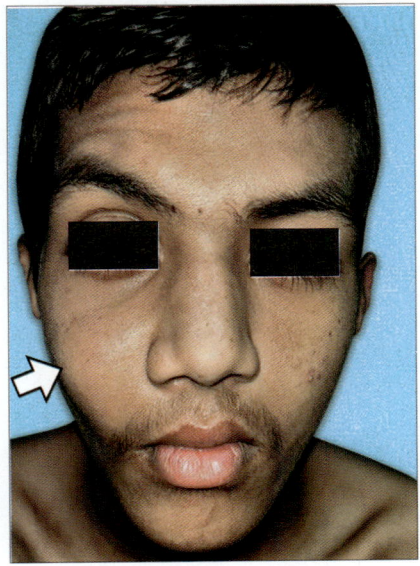

Q9. The following image shows a 53-year-old lady with right sided facial swelling, pain, nasal obstruction and blood-stained nasal discharge. There is also mass present in the nasal cavity.
   a. What is the most probable diagnosis?
   b. What is the extent of the Ohngren's line?
   c. What is the significance of Ohngren's line?

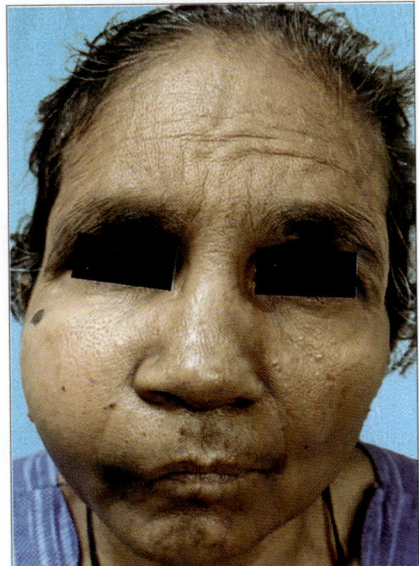

Q10. The following image shows a 55-year-old lady with a huge, non-tender swelling in the frontal region developing over 1 year. Imaging confirmed a cystic swelling involving the frontal and ethmoidal sinuses, causing displacement of the orbit.

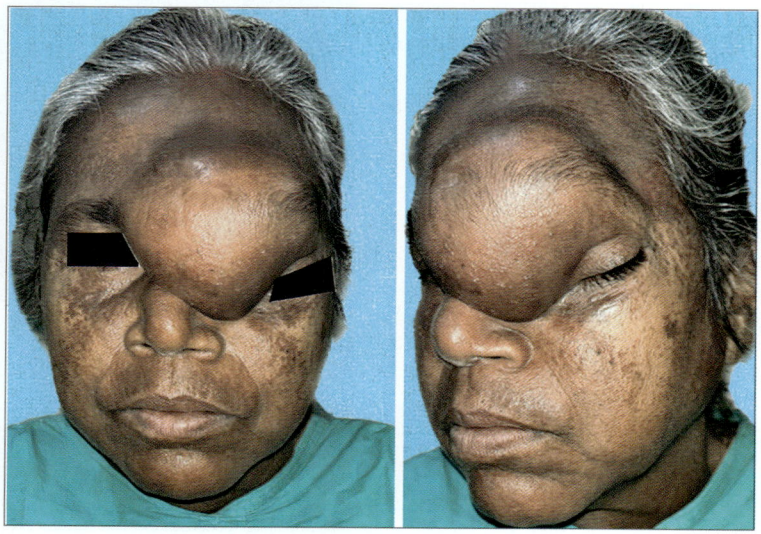

  a. What is the most probable diagnosis?
  b. What is the most common sinus to be involved in this entity?
  c. What is the treatment you will do?

Q11. The following diagram shows the complications of sinusitis:

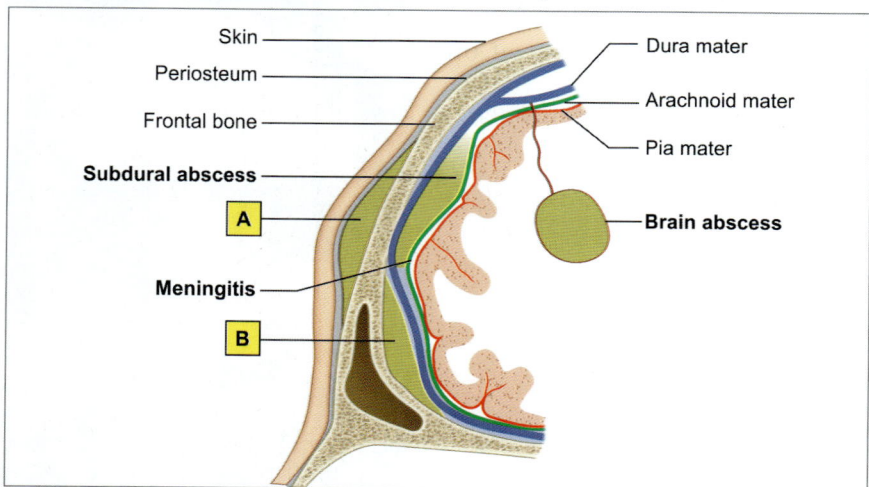

  a. What are the two complications marked as 'A' and 'B' in the diagram above?
  b. What is the key point of difference between orbital apex syndrome and superior orbital fissure syndrome?
  c. Mention two symptoms of cavernous sinus thrombosis.

Q12. The following is showing an image of a firm swelling in the nasal cavity. It is non-tender, progressively increasing in size. It was seen to originate from the septum. It was posted for excision after investigations.

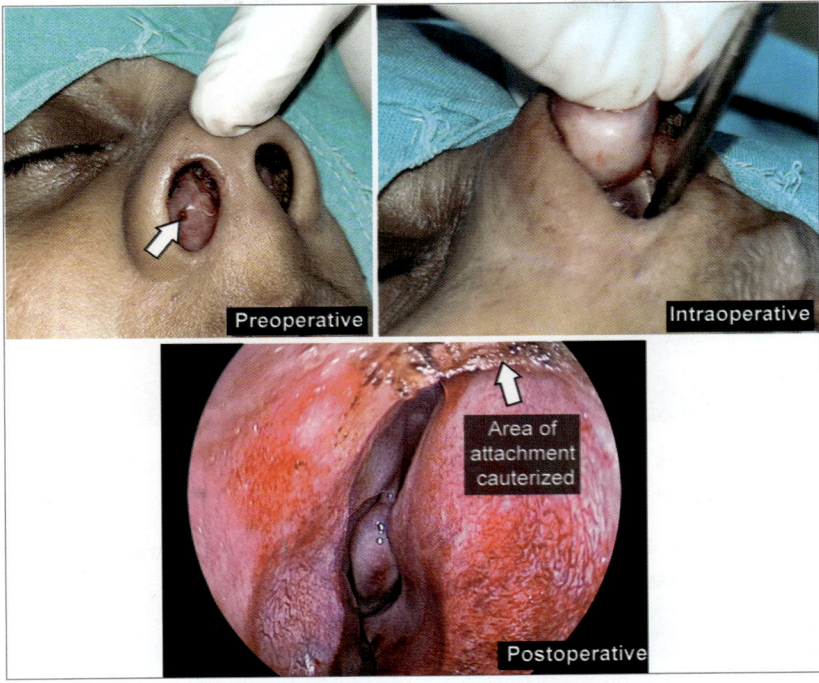

a. Give 2 differentials for such nasal masses arising from the nasal septum.
b. What imaging will you order for the patient before planning for excision?
c. What is the origin of esthesioneuroblastoma?

Q13. The following image is of the vestibule of a 38-year-old gentleman, with this swelling inside:

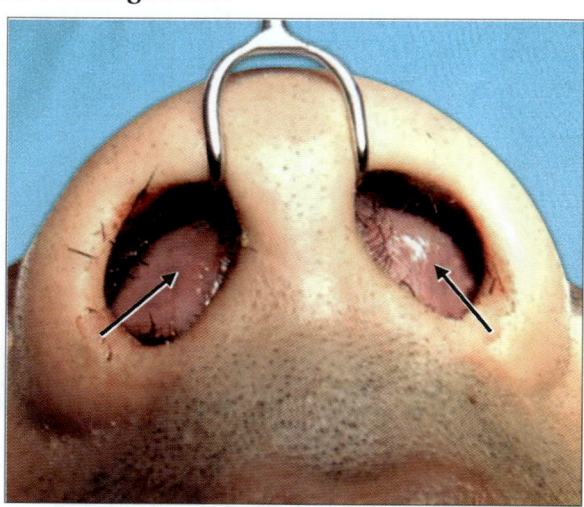

a. What is the most probable diagnosis from the picture shown above?
b. What is the treatment of choice?

Q14. This is a 40-year-old gentleman with an unilateral polypoidal nasal mass, with occasional history of epistaxis:

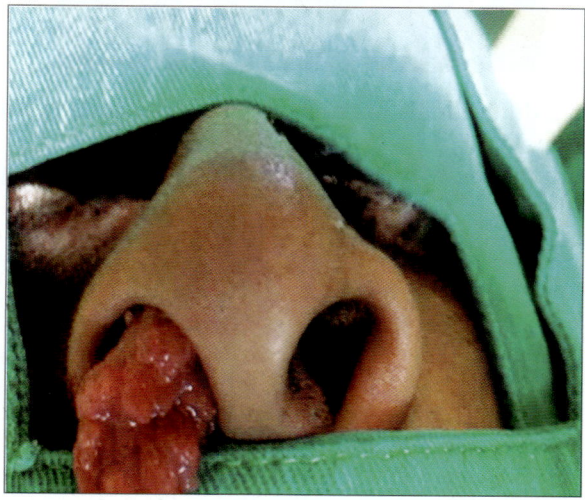

a. What is the diagnosis shown in the picture?
b. Name the pathogen causing it.
c. What is the treatment?

CHAPTER 9: Clinical Methods 67

Q15. The following photographs are of a 13-year-old boy with a history of epistaxis and nasal mass.

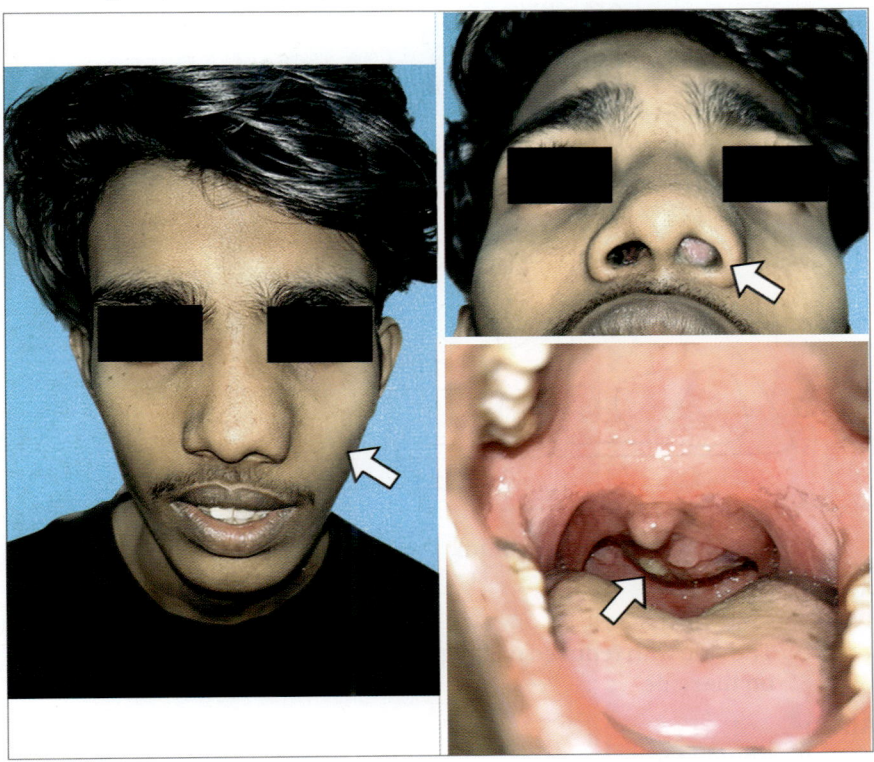

a. What is the facies being shown in the picture above?
b. Name the disease which most commonly causes the facies?
c. Name two investigations to be ordered for this patient.

ANSWERS

Ans 1:
   a. Anterior rhinoscopy
   b. Labelled diagram of anterior rhinoscopy:

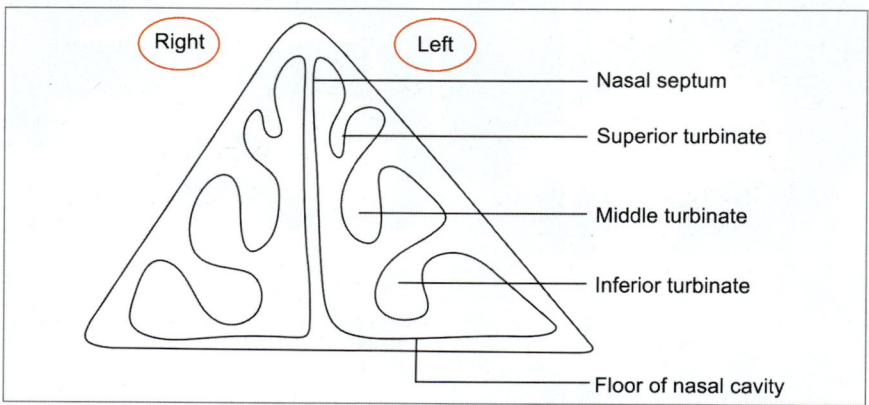

   c. Thudicum's nasal speculum

Ans 2:
   a. Cold spatula test
   b. The side with reduced misting signifies that there is nasal obstruction on that side

Ans 3:
   a. Cottle's test
   b. True
   c. Internal nasal valve area

Ans 4:
   a. Cotton-wool test
   b. In case of nasal obstruction due to polyp/septum deviation, the movement of the cotton fluff on that side would be reduced

Ans 5:
   a. Paranasal sinus tenderness
   b. Acute sinusitis

Ans 6:
a. Posterior rhinoscopy
b. Labelled diagram of posterior rhinoscopy:

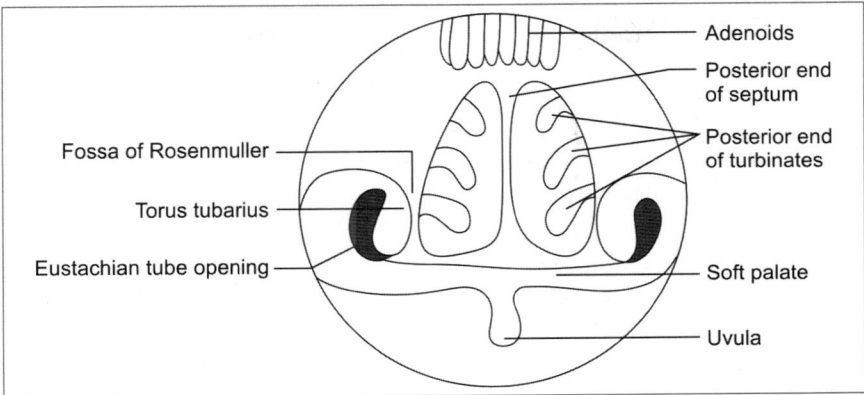

Ans 7:
a. 'A': Closed nasal bone fracture reduction using elevator
'B': Closed septal reduction
b. Asch's septal forceps
c. Presence of edema interferes with accurate reduction by closed methods. Thus, the best time to reduce is before the appearance of edema or after it has subsided which is usually in 5–7 days

Ans 8:
a. i. Fibrous dysplasia
ii. Ossifying fibroma
b. NCCT nose and paranasal sinuses
c. Odontogenic tissue

Ans 9:
a. Carcinoma of the maxillary sinus
b. Ohngren's line extends from the medial canthus of the eye to the angle of the mandible
c. Growths posterosuperior to this line (suprastructural) have a poorer prognosis than those anteroinferior to it (infrastructural)

Ans 10:
a. Fronto-ethmoidal mucocele
b. Frontal sinus: Most common paranasal sinus to be involved by mucocele
c. Frontal sinusotomy with ethmoidectomy (by endoscopic, external or combined approach) with free drainage of the frontal sinus into the middle meatus

SECTION 2: Nose and Paranasal Sinuses

Ans 11:
  a. A: Pott's puffy tumor (osteomyelitis of the frontal bone)
     B: Extradural abscess
  b. Involvement of cranial nerve II (optic nerve) leading to vision loss occurs in orbital apex syndrome, not in superior orbital fissure syndrome
  c. i. Total ophthalmoplegia (due to cranial nerves III, IV, VI being involved)
     ii. Diminution of sensation in the distribution of V1 (ophthalmic division of trigeminal nerve)

Ans 12:
  a. Nasal septal hemangioma, squamous papilloma
  b. CECT (nose + paranasal sinus)—as suspicion of hemangioma/malignant mass is present
  c. Olfactory epithelium (in the upper third of the nose)

Ans 13:
  a. Septal hematoma
  b. Incision, drainage and suction

Ans 14:
  a. Rhinosporidiosis
  b. *Rhinosporidium seeberi*
  c. Complete surgical excision, cauterization of base

Ans 15:
  a. Frog face deformity
  b. Juvenile nasopharyngeal angiofibroma (JNA)
  c. i. CECT nose, paranasal sinuses with CT angiography
     ii. MRI face, nose and paranasal sinuses

CHAPTER 10

Surgical Procedures

Q1. The following image shows the incisions used in septoplasty:

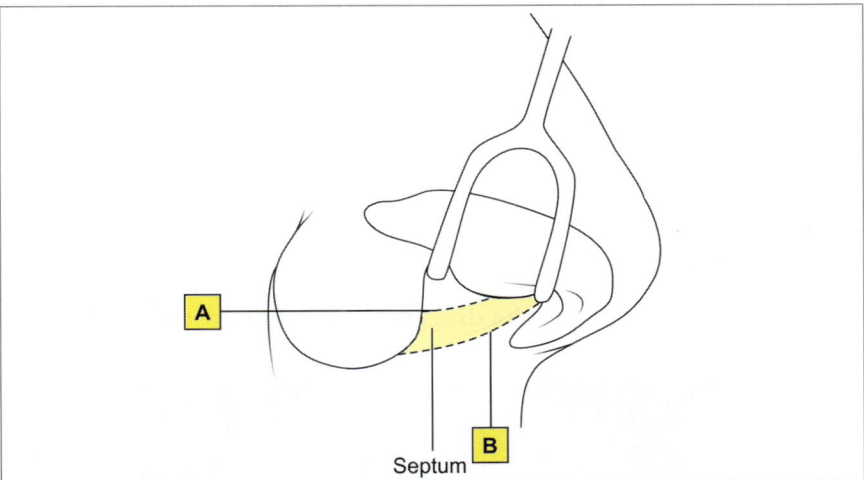

a. What are the names of the incision marked by 'A' and 'B'?
b. What is the dose of (lignocaine + adrenaline) that is used for local infiltration?
c. Name 2 corrective methods used in septoplasty.

Q2. The following image shows a step being performed in septoplasty:

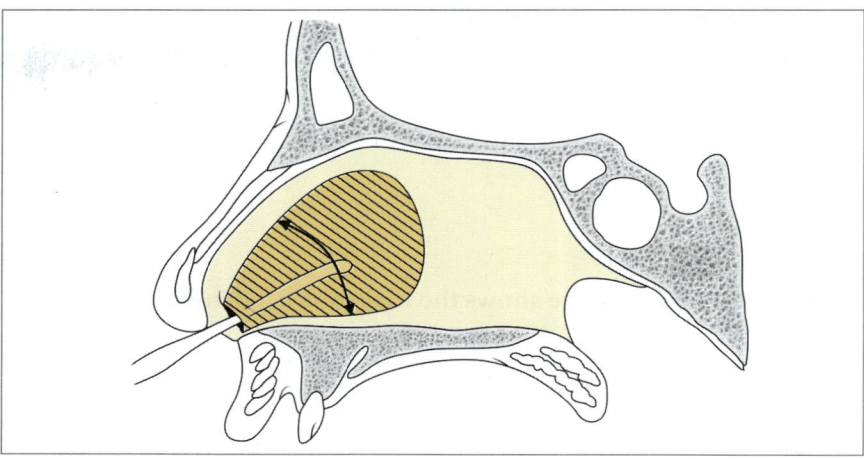

a. What is the step being performed?
b. Name the instrument that is generally used for this step.
c. How much of the septal cartilage should be left intact in submucosal resection (SMR) surgery to maintain tip and dorsal nasal support?

Q3. The following shows the diagnostic nasal endoscopy photo of a patient:

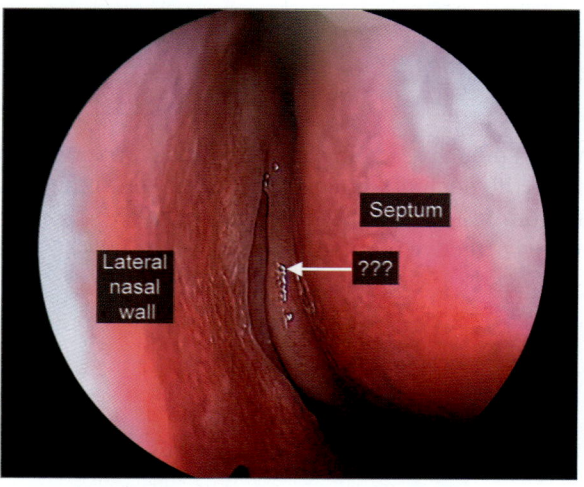

a. What is the structure being asked in the photo above?
b. What are the structures seen on the first pass during DNE?
c. How is the nose prepared for DNE?

CHAPTER 10: Surgical Procedures

Q4. The following is an endoscopic image following functional endoscopic sinus surgery (FESS):

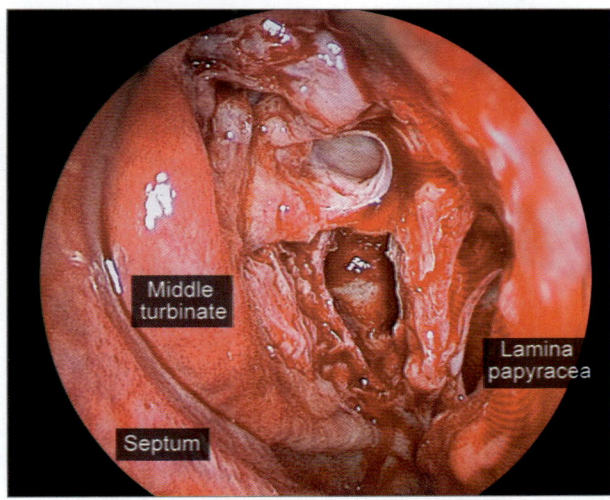

a. Mention two complications of FESS.
b. What is the ideal position of the patient during FESS?
c. What is (i) Stammberger's technique, (ii) Wigand's technique in FESS?

Q5. Observe the photo:

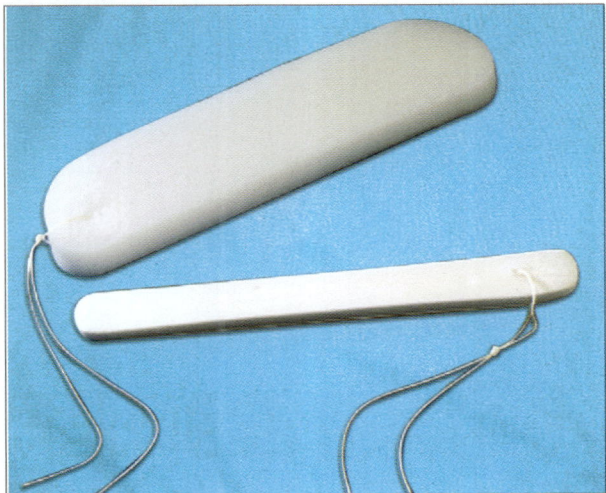

a. What is the image showing?
b. What is it used for?
c. Give 2 indications for its use.

Q6. The following image is showing a 9-year-old boy who has come with the history of insertion of a plastic bead inside the left nose.

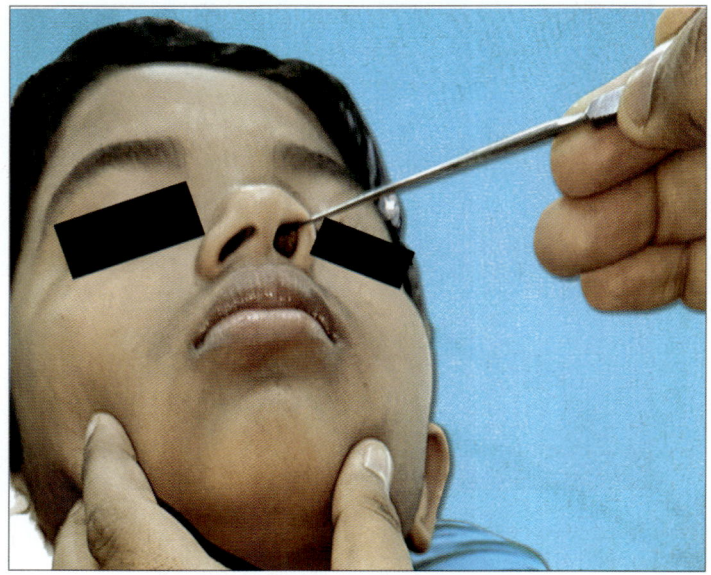

a. What is the procedure being performed here?
b. What is the instrument used for this?
c. Mention two complications that can occur in this procedure.

Q7. A 62-year-old male, known hypertensive on irregular medications, presented with nasal bleeding to the ENT emergency. The following intervention was done on the patient:

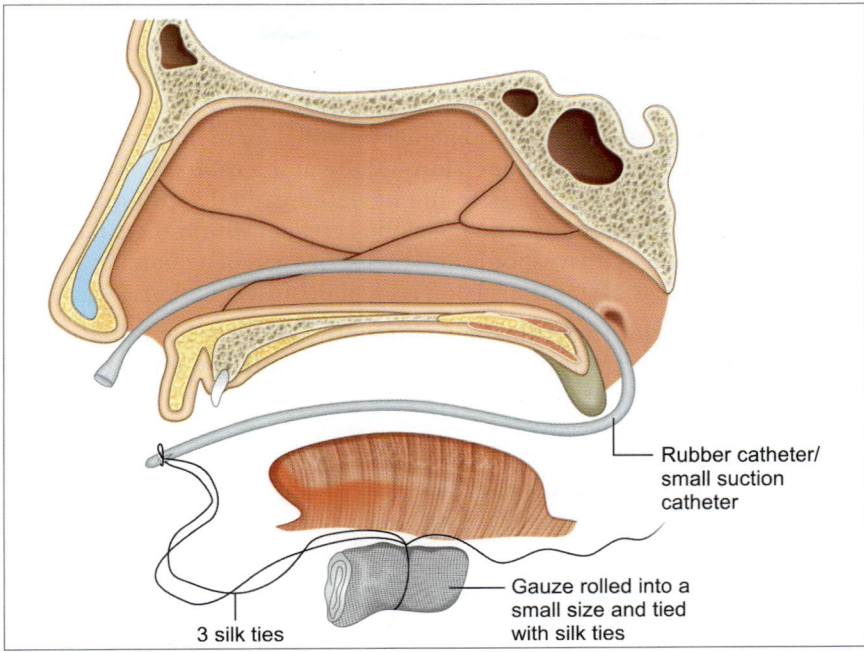

a. What was the procedure done in the patient?
b. What can be used alternatively to do this?

ANSWERS

Ans 1:
   a. **'A': Killian's incision**—Created approximately 1 to 2 cm posterior to the caudal septal margin within the respiratory epithelium. Useful when septal deviation is only in the middle to the posterior third of the nasal cavity. Greatest downfall is in its relative inaccessibility to the caudal septal edge, and higher potential for membrane tearing
'B': Hemi-transfixion incision—Made at the caudal border of the septum allowing access to the deviated caudal septum and any posterior deflections. The incision is created within the squamous epithelium of the vestibule and hence has less of a tendency to tear under stress. Hemi-transfixion is ideal in most situations

      ** Transfixion/full-transfixion incision—Similar to hemi-transfixion and then accomplished by incising completely through to the opposite membrane

   b. 7 mg/kg body weight
   c. 2 corrective methods:
      i. Scoring on the concave side
      ii. Shaving on the convex side

Ans 2:
   a. Elevation of the mucoperichondrial flap through the subperichondrial pocket
   b. Freer's elevator
   c. At a minimum, a 1 cm dorsal and caudal segment should be left intact (L-strut)

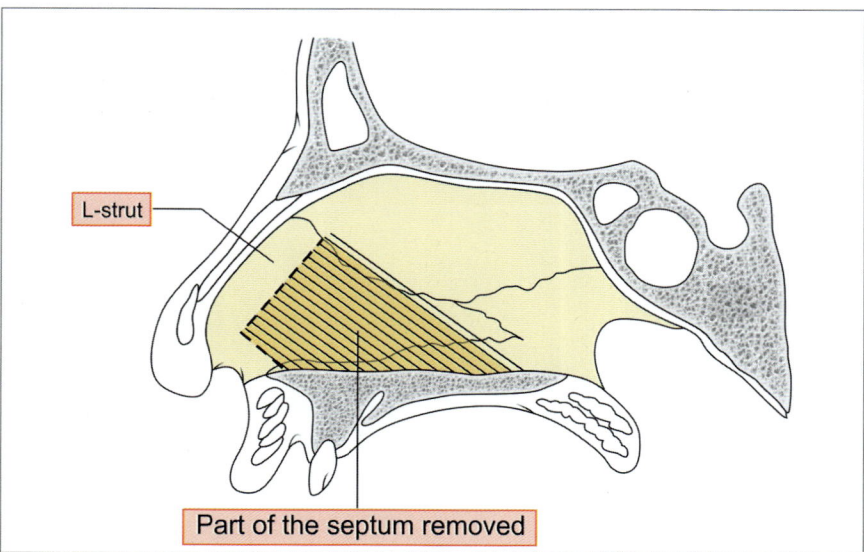

Ans 3:
a. Middle turbinate (right)
b. Inferior meatus, inferior turbinate, floor of nasal cavity, nasopharynx (in detail)
c. Nasal spray/drops: Xylometazoline (0.1%)
   Nasal packs soaked with 4% topical anesthetic (lignocaine) and adrenaline (1:1000)

Ans 4:
a. Orbital hematoma, CSF rhinorrhea
b. Supine, head-end elevated 15°–30°
c. (i) Stammberger's technique: Anterior to posterior
   (ii) Wigand's technique: Posterior to anterior

Ans 5:
a. Merocel nasal pack
b. Anterior nasal packing
c. (i) Anterior epistaxis
   (ii) Nasal packing after nasal surgeries

Ans 6:
a. Foreign body removal
b. Foreign body hook
c. 2 complications:
   i. Bleeding from the nose
   ii. Foreign body getting impacted in the adenoid tissue of child

Ans 7:
a. Posterior nasal packing
b. Foley's catheter, inflating the bulb in the nasopharynx to stop bleeders there

Development

Q1. The following diagram shows the embryological development of the primitive nose and palate:

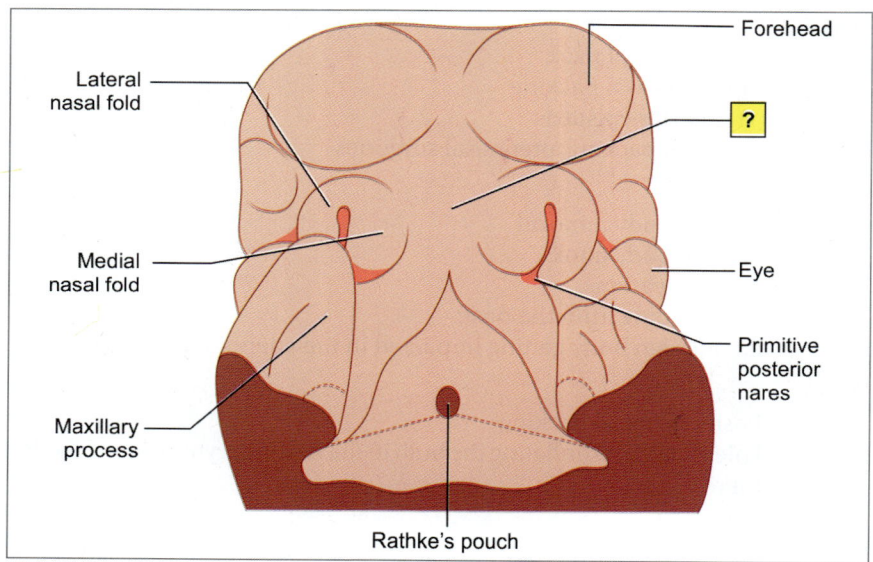

a. When does the facial development begin?
b. What is the structure being asked in the diagram above?
c. Name two structures of the face formed by it.
d. Failure of breakdown of the bucconasal membrane during embryological development leads what pathology?

Q2. The following is showing the CT scan of the paranasal sinuses of a 6-year-old girl. Answer the following about development of the paranasal sinuses:

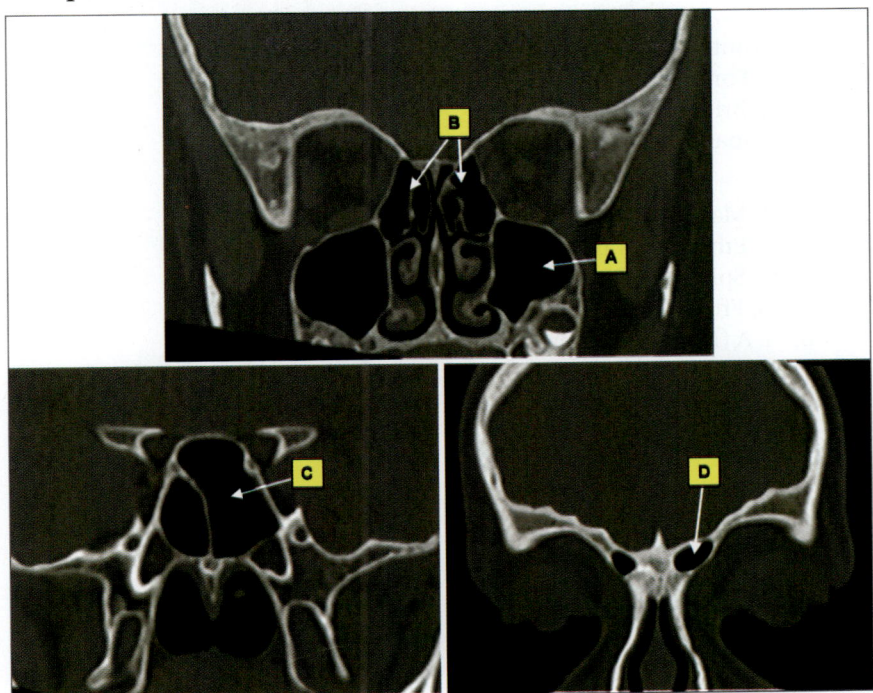

a. Name the sinuses A/ B/ C/ D as marked in the CT images.
b. Which sinus among these A/ B/ C/ D, is the ----
   (i) First to develop
   (ii) Last to develop
c. Which of these sinuses ---- A/ B/ C/ D, are ----
   (i) Present at birth
   (ii) Absent at birth

ANSWERS

Ans 1:
- a. 4th week of gestation (intra-uterine life)
- b. Fronto-nasal process
- c. i. Forehead
   ii. Bridge of nose
- d. Choanal atresia

Ans 2:
- a. A: Maxillary sinus
   B: Ethmoid sinus
   C: Sphenoid sinus
   D: Frontal sinus
- b. i. A (Maxillary sinus is the first sinus to develop)
   ii. D (Frontal sinus is the last sinus to develop)
- c. i. A/B (Maxillary and ethmoid sinuses are present at birth)
   ii. C/D (Frontal and sphenoid sinuses are absent at birth)

SECTION 3

THROAT

Section Outline

12. Oral Cavity
13. Salivary Glands
14. Pharynx and Esophagus
15. Larynx and Trachea

Oral Cavity

Q1. The following photograph is of a lesion on the right side of the floor of the mouth:

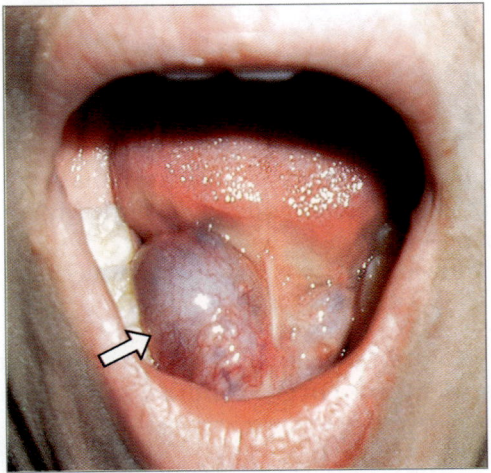

a. What is the diagnosis?
b. What is the treatment of choice?
c. What is it known as when the lesion extends into the neck?

Q2. A 38-year-old gentleman developed this ulcerative lesion on the tongue over 1 month:

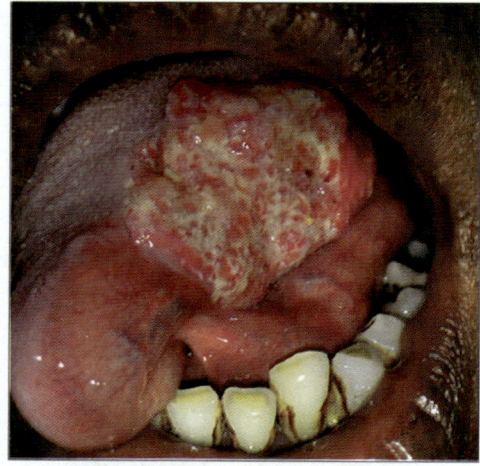

a. What is the most common site of carcinoma in the tongue?
b. Bilateral/contralateral node involvement is common in tongue carcinoma—True/False.
c. Pain in the ipsilateral ear is a common finding in carcinoma tongue—why?

Q3. A 56-year-old man developed an ulcero-proliferative lesion on the left buccal mucosa over 2 months:

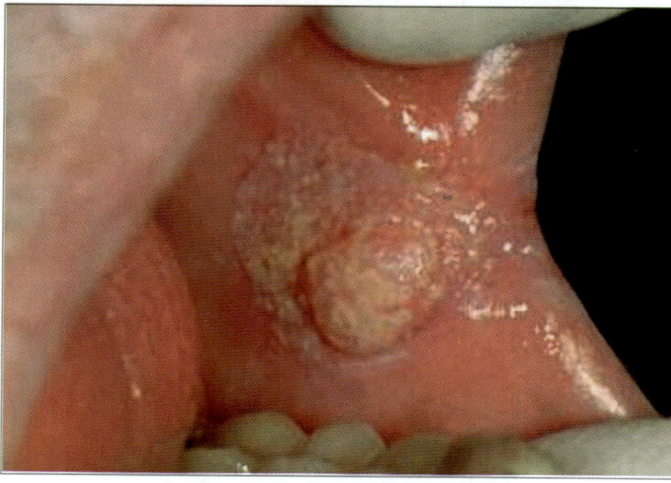

a. What is the most common histologic type of buccal mucosa carcinoma?
b. What investigation will you order for this patient, to help in disease staging?
c. Name two etiological factors, for carcinoma buccal mucosa.

Q4. A 33-year-old man develops recurrent superficial ulcers on the lip and other parts of the oral cavity, which heals in a few days.

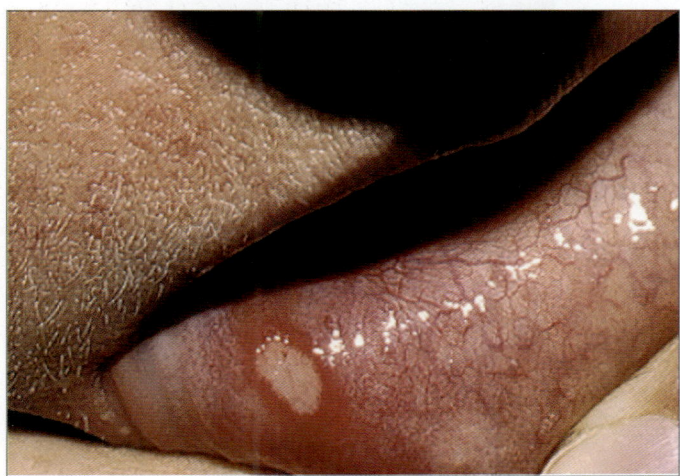

  a. What is the diagnosis?
  b. What is the treatment?

Q5. The following image shows an examination procedure:

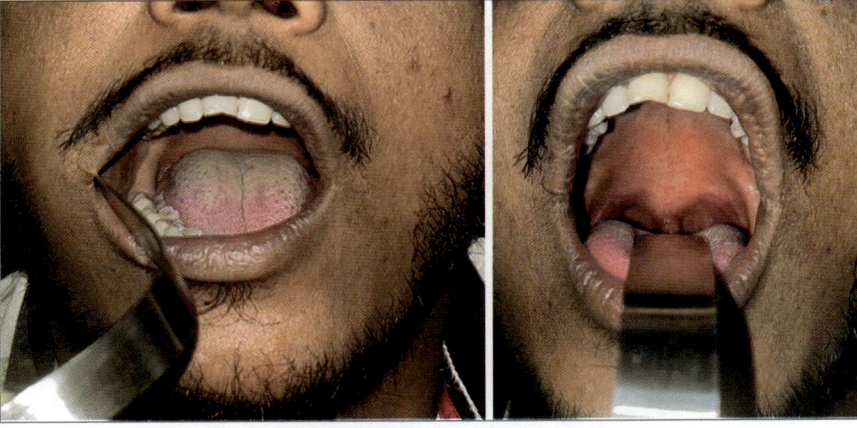

  a. What is the examination being performed?
  b. What is the instrument being used?
  c. Name 3 clinical findings to look for in the hard palate during this procedure.

Q6. The following photograph is of a 26-year-old male with a history of recurrent swelling on the lower lip as shown:

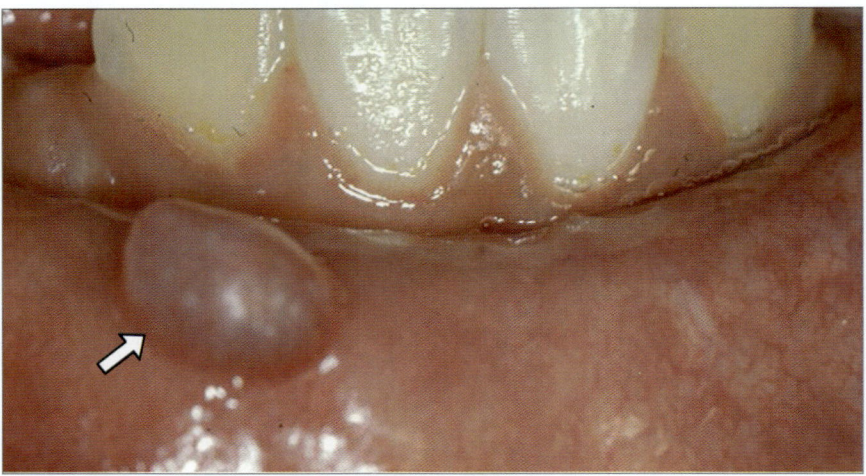

a. What is the diagnosis?
b. What is the origin of these cystic lesions?
c. What is the treatment?

Q7. A 22-year-old lady presented with the complaints of a reddish lesion on the lateral part of the lip on the left side, with history of intermittent bleeding and increase in size.

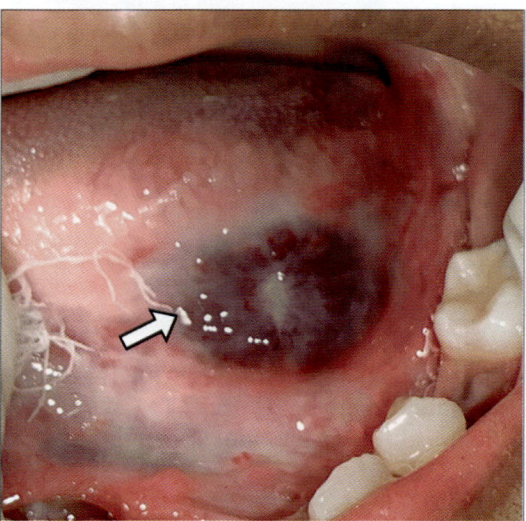

a. What is the most probable diagnosis?
b. What are the two main types?
c. Name 2 treatment modalities for this entity.

Q8. The following image shows a lesion on the right angle of mouth in a 33-year-old male smoker developing over 1 year.

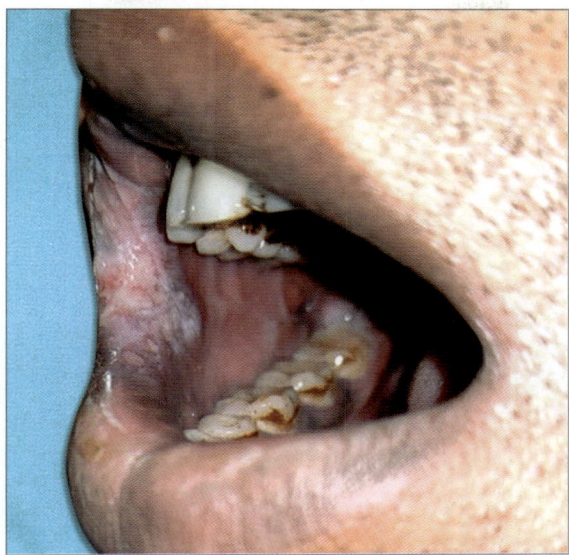

a. What is the most probable diagnosis?
b. What are its 3 types?
c. Why is biopsy indicated in this patient?

Q9. Oral sub-mucosal fibrosis is widely seen in India due to the habit of betel-nut chewing. With respect to that, answer the following:

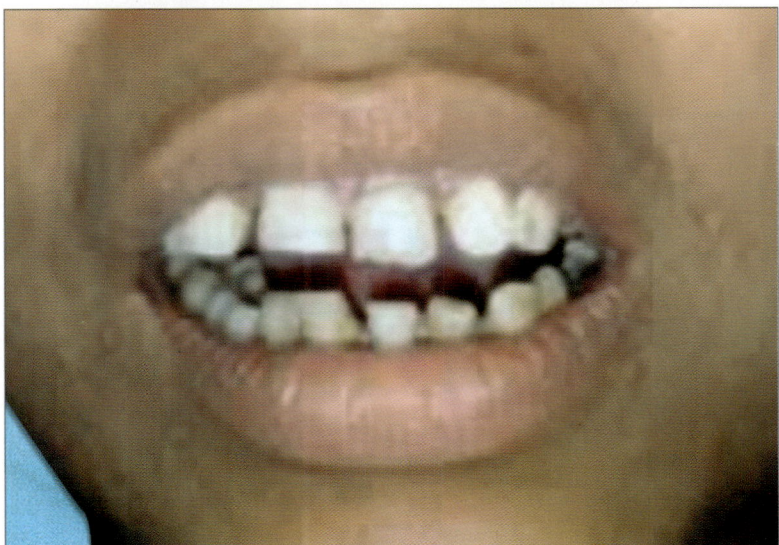

a. Two symptoms of the disease.
b. What finding can be appreciated on palpation of the oral cavity?
c. What is the medical treatment for the condition?

SECTION 3: Throat

Q10. The patient came with the complaint of eruption of clusters of multiple vesicles, with fever:

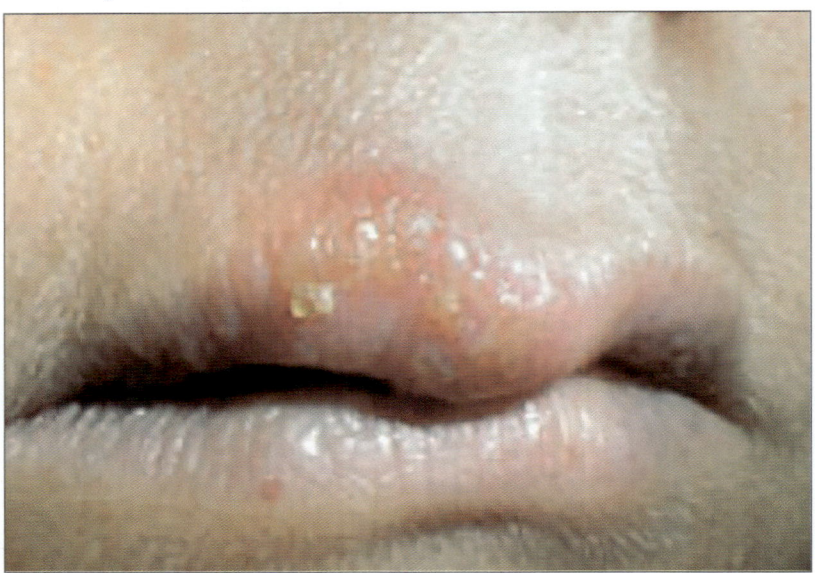

a. What is the diagnosis from the photo above?
b. What is the treatment you will administer?

Q11. A 38-year-old diabetic man, developed the following lesions in the oral cavity which could not be scraped off.

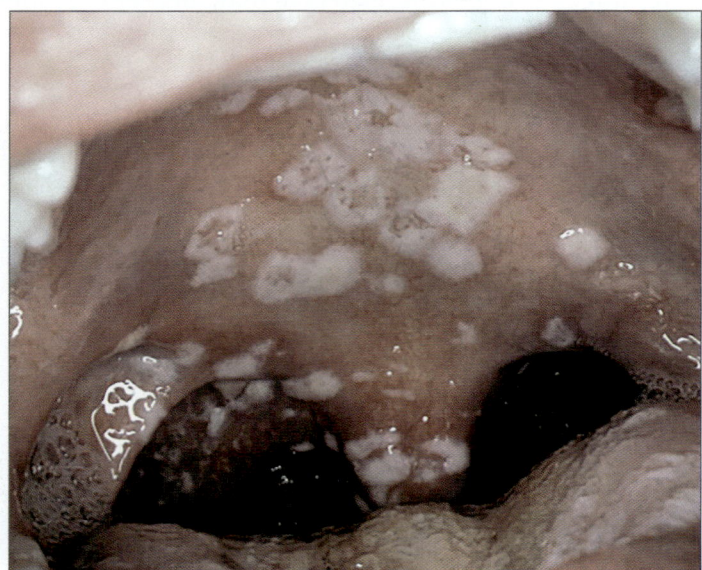

a. What is the most probable diagnosis?
b. What treatment will you administer?

Q12. The following shows a proliferative lesion over the hard palate in a 55-year-old male:

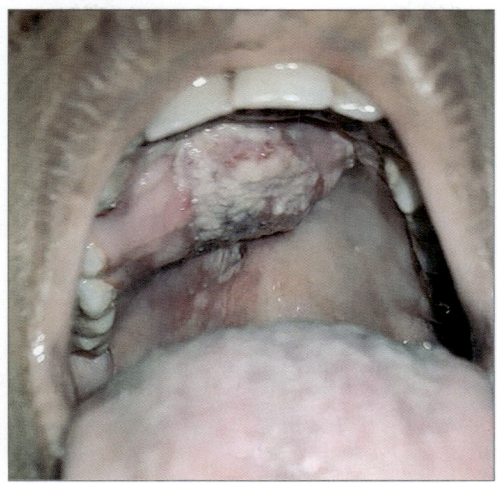

  a. What is the most common location of minor salivary gland neoplasms in general?
  b. What is the most common type of minor salivary gland neoplasms?
  c. What imaging modality will you order for this patient now? (Name 1)

Q13. A 13-year-boy came with difficulty in articulation of some words while speaking. The following was found on examination:

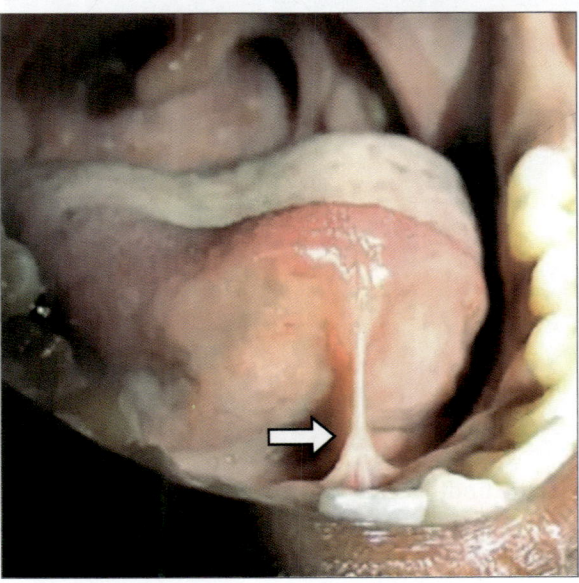

  a. What is being shown by the arrow in the photograph?
  b. What is restriction of tongue mobility known as?
  c. What is the treatment you will initially give to this boy?

Q14. The patient presented with the following appearance of the tongue, with complaints of burning sensation while eating.

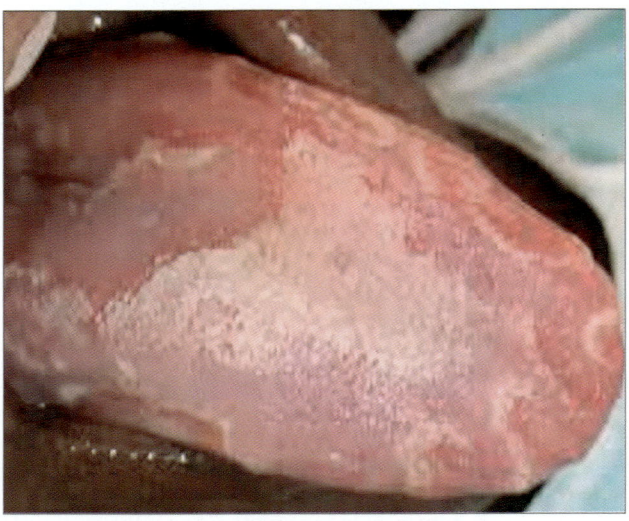

  a. What is the diagnosis from the photograph above?
  b. What treatment can you give the patient?

Q15. The following is showing a 60-year-old male who presented to the ENT OPD with the following finding:

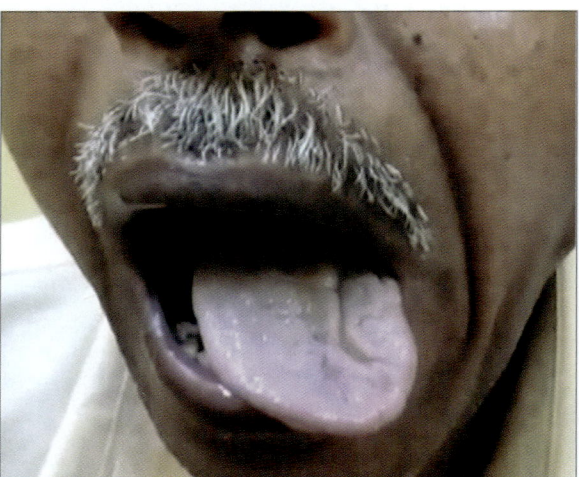

  a. What is the finding shown in the picture above?
  b. Name one clinical condition/pathology in which the above finding can be present?

CHAPTER 12: Oral Cavity

ANSWERS

Ans 1:
  a. Ranula
  b. Complete surgical excision (if small), marsupialization (if large)
  c. Plunging ranula

Ans 2:
  a. Lateral border (middle or ventral part)
  b. True
  c. Referred pain due to common nerve supply – tongue (lingual nerve) and ear (auriculo-temporal nerve) – both from mandibular division of trigeminal nerve

Ans 3:
  a. Squamous cell carcinoma
  b. Contrast enhanced CT scan of face and neck (base of skull to T4)
  c. Smoking, alcohol

Ans 4:
  a. Aphthous ulcers
  b. Treatment: Topical steroid applications, local pain relieved with lignocaine viscous

Ans 5:
  a. Examination of the oral cavity and oropharynx
  b. Lack's tongue depressor
  c. 3 findings in the hard palate:
     i. Cleft palate
     ii. Oronasal fistula
     iii. High-arched palate

Ans 6:
  a. Mucocele
  b. Minor salivary glands of lower lip
  c. Complete surgical excision

Ans 7:
  a. Hemangioma (of tongue)
  b. i. Capillary hemangioma
     ii. Cavernous hemangioma
  c. Sclerotherapy, laser

Ans 8:
  a. Leukoplakia
  b. i. Homogeneous, ii. Nodular (speckled), iii. Erythroleukoplakia
  c. To rule out malignancy. On an average 5% become malignant

Ans 9:
- a. i. Intolerance to spicy food, burning sensation, soreness of mouth
     ii. Difficulty in opening mouth (trismus)
- b. Fibrotic bands can be palpated in the affected areas
- c. Medical treatment: Topical injection of steroids (e.g., Dexamethasone 1 mL) along with hyaluronic acid (1500 IU), in the affected area, biweekly for 8–10 weeks – relieves trismus and brings improvement

Ans 10:
- a. Herpes labialis
- b. Symptomatic treatment. Tab. Acyclovir (200 mg)—5 times a day for 5 days helps reduce recurrence

Ans 11:
- a. Oral thrush (candidiasis)—caused by *Candida albicans*
- b. Treatment: By topical application of nystatin or clotrimazole, oral antifungal medications may be given

Ans 12:
- a. Site of predilection: Soft or hard palate
- b. Pleomorphic salivary adenoma
- c. CECT face + neck (base of skull to T4)

Ans 13:
- a. Tongue tie
- b. Ankyloglossia
- c. Speech therapy (as the boy is having difficulty in articulation of certain words only, it is unlikely that it is due the presence of tongue-tie. Not every tongue-tie needs to be released. If the tongue can be protruded beyond the lower incisors, it is unlikely to cause any speech defects)

Ans 14:
- a. Geographical tongue
- b. Medical management with multivitamin tablets, dietary modifications

Ans 15:
- a. Hypoglossal nerve palsy (left)
- b. Infarct affecting hypoglossal nucleus, Schwannoma/paraganglioma, metastatic deposits at skull base, sarcoidosis, etc.

CHAPTER 13

Salivary Glands

Q1. The following diagram shows some neck spaces:

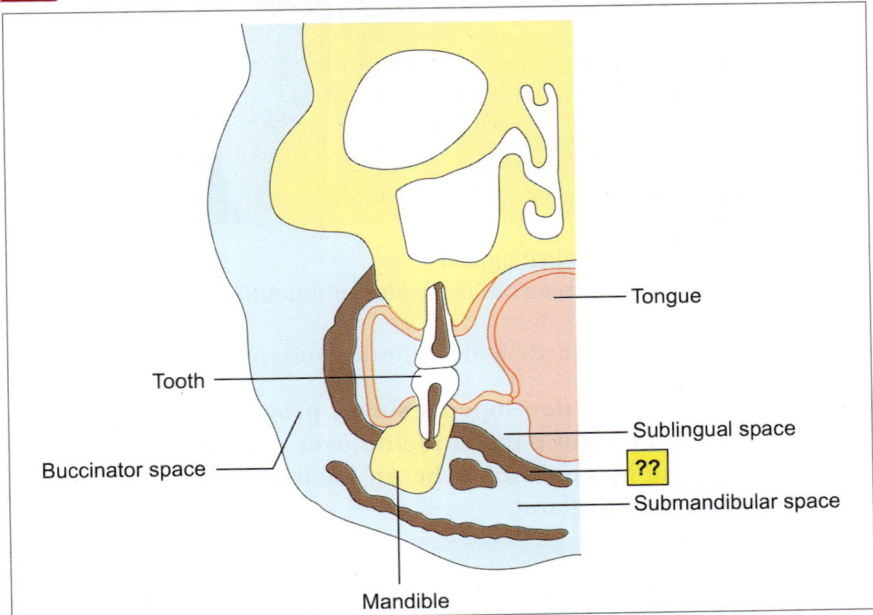

a. What is the muscle being asked in the diagram above?
b. Which part of the oral cavity does that muscle primarily form?
c. Name the condition where there is acute infection of the spaces shown in the diagram.
d. What is the most common cause of this acute infection?

Q2. The following photograph shows of a 25-year-old lady with complaint of intermittent swelling and pain on the submandibular region on the right side:

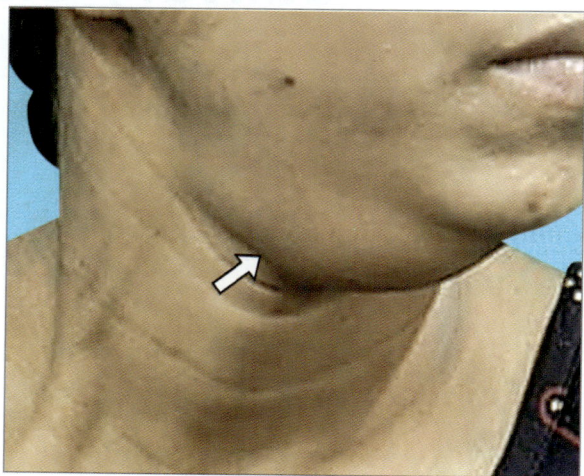

a. What is the probable diagnosis?
b. What investigation can be advised for submandibular salivary calculi detection?
c. Name two antibodies helping in the diagnosis of Sjogren's syndrome.

Q3. A 48-year-old man developed a slowly progressive, non-tender swelling on the right parotid region over one and a half years. Ultrasonography confirms it be an enlargement of superficial lobe of the parotid gland.

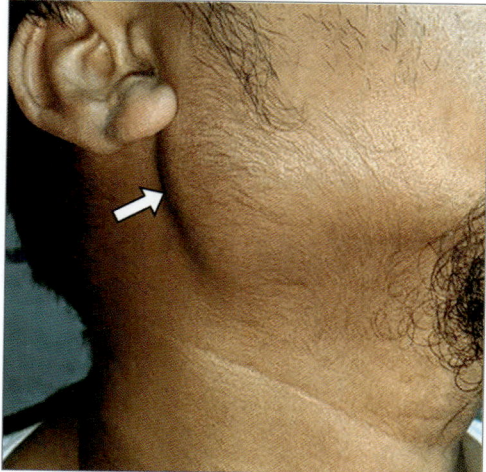

a. What is the most common benign tumor of the salivary glands?
b. Name 2 histologic types of malignant tumors of salivary glands.
c. What are the 5 features that indicate malignant transformation in a benign salivary gland tumor, clinically?

CHAPTER 13: Salivary Glands

ANSWERS

Ans 1:
- a. Mylohyoid muscle
- b. Floor of mouth
- c. Ludwig's angina – (Acute infection of bilateral sublingual, submandibular and submental spaces, gross edema of the floor of mouth and anterior tongue)
- d. Dental infection

Ans 2:
- a. Submandibular sialadenitis
- b. Digital X-ray soft tissue lateral neck (to pick up radio-opaque stones), sialography may be required for radiolucent stones
- c. SS-A and SS-B antibodies

Ans 3:
- a. Pleomorphic adenoma ("mixed tumors")
- b.
  - i. Mucoepidermoid carcinoma
  - ii. Adenoid cystic carcinoma (has characteristic perineural spread and VII nerve involvement)
- c.
  - i. Rapid growth
  - ii. Pain
  - iii. Paresthesia
  - iv. Fixity and involvement of overlying skin
  - v. Palsy (VII nerve or others)

Pharynx and Esophagus

Q1. The following diagram shows the structures in the tonsillar bed:

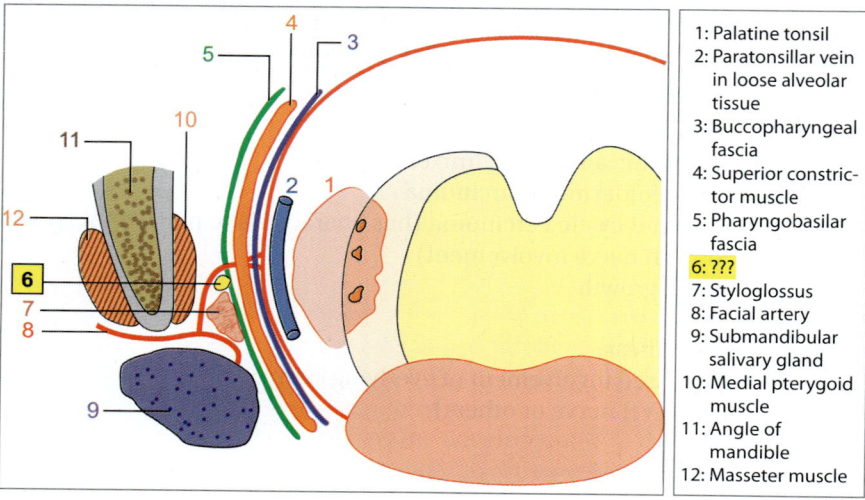

1: Palatine tonsil
2: Paratonsillar vein in loose alveolar tissue
3: Buccopharyngeal fascia
4: Superior constrictor muscle
5: Pharyngobasilar fascia
6: ???
7: Styloglossus
8: Facial artery
9: Submandibular salivary gland
10: Medial pterygoid muscle
11: Angle of mandible
12: Masseter muscle

a. What is the structure marked number '6'?
b. Any pathology affecting the tonsils or tonsillar fossa may present as pain referred to the ear. What is the possible explanation of this?
c. Mention 3 arteries supplying the tonsil.

CHAPTER 14: Pharynx and Esophagus   97

Q2. The following photograph is of a 17-year-old boy suffering from recurrent throat infections:

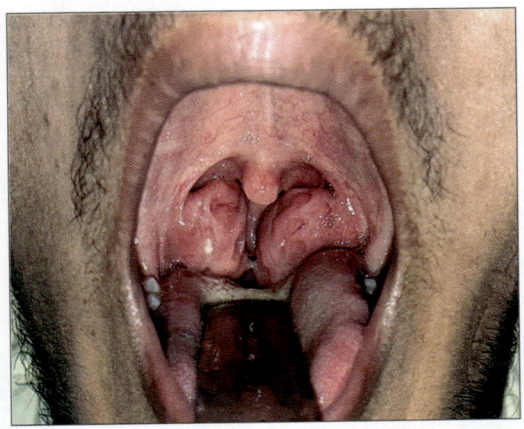

a. What is the grade of tonsillar hypertrophy in this patient?
b. Mention 3 complications of chronic tonsillitis.
c. Monospot test (modification of Paul Bunnell test) was done previously in this patient. What was the probable diagnosis to rule out, for which the test was done?
d. Name a surgery in which tonsil is removed as a part of the procedure.

Q3. The following shows a nasal endoscopic photograph:

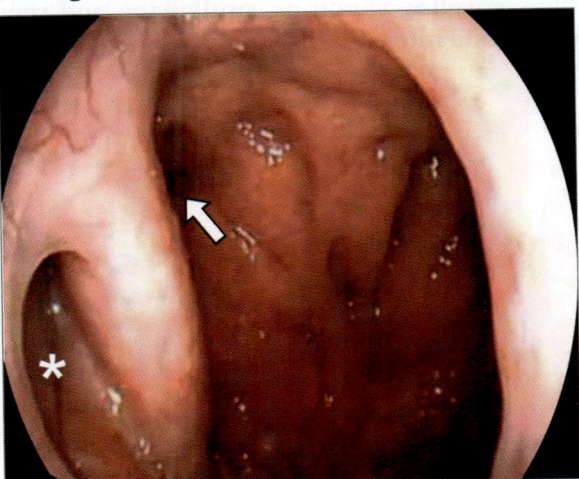

a. What is the region shown in the picture?
b. Name the structures marked with: (i) White arrow (ii) Star mark
c. What is the most common presentation of a cancer of the region shown?

Q4. This is a fiberoptic laryngoscopy photograph of a 72-year-old male with foreign body sensation in throat and intermittent pain:

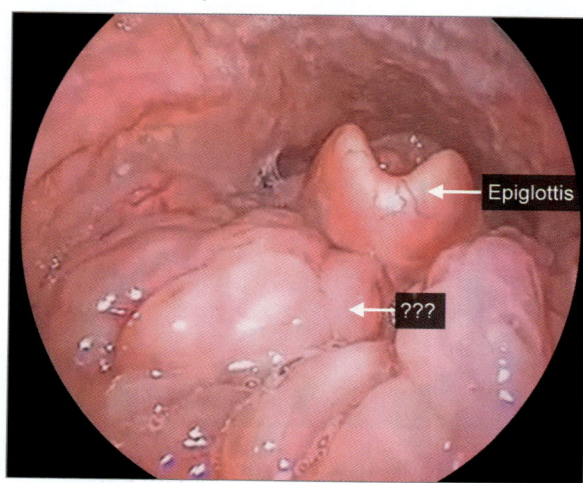

a. What is being shown in the photograph by question marks?
b. What are the subsites of the oropharynx?
c. What is the most common histologic variety of cancers of the oropharynx?

Q5. The following diagrams show a condition where there is dysphagia, gurgling sound on swallowing and regurgitation of undigested food intermittently.

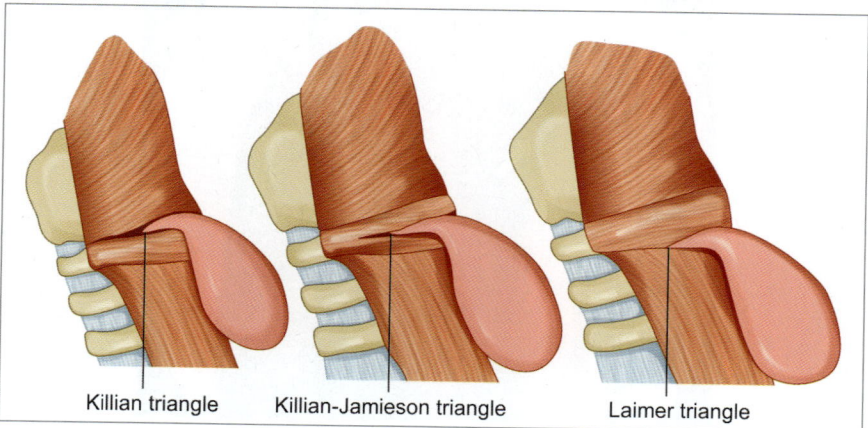

a. What is the diagnosis?
b. What is the investigation you will order primarily?
c. What is the treatment?

Q6. The following is a photograph of a 7-year-old boy with complaints of decreased scholastic performance, snoring and open-mouth breathing:

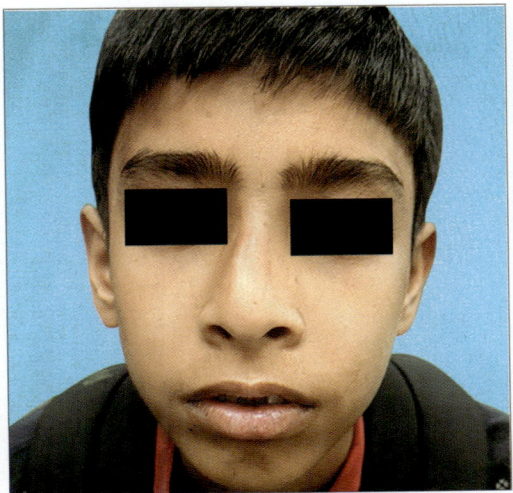

a. What is the most probable diagnosis?
b. What is the initial treatment you will give to the patient?
c. Name one investigation you will advise this patient to get done.

Q7. The following image is of a boy, aged 12 years, who presented to the ENT OPD with complaints of open mouth breathing, snoring and decreased hearing:

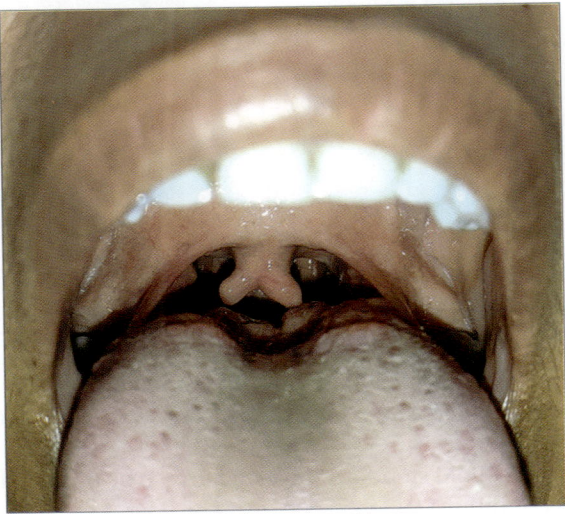

a. What is the finding shown in the photograph?
b. What other clinical entity can it be associated with?
c. What is the risk associated with adenoidectomy in such patients?

Q8. The following shows the photograph of a 22-year-old male with history of recurrent throat infections. He also has addiction history of excessive smoking and alcohol consumption.

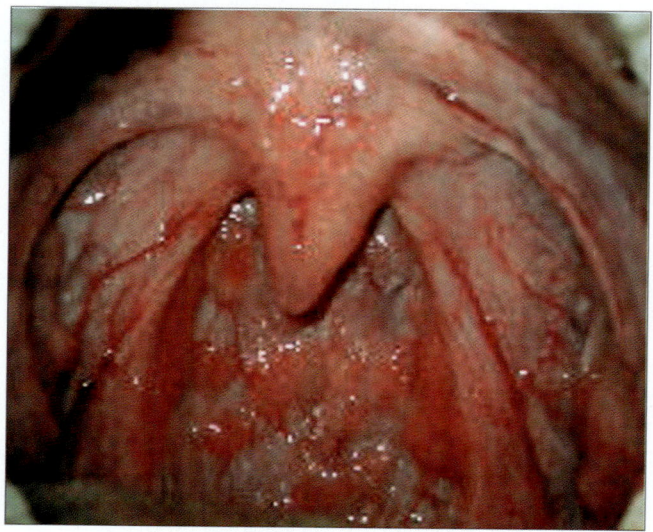

a. What is the most probable diagnosis?
b. Give two symptoms that this patient will have?

Q9. Observe the illustrations below.

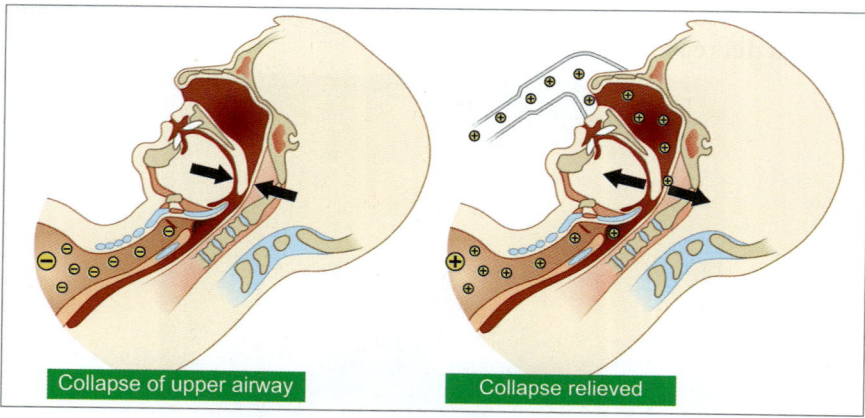

a. What is the being shown in the illustration above?
b. Name the clinical entity for which it is used as a treatment modality primarily.
c. What is the "gold standard" investigation to be ordered for diagnosis of this condition?
d. What is DISE?

Q10. With regard to the esophagus, answer the following:

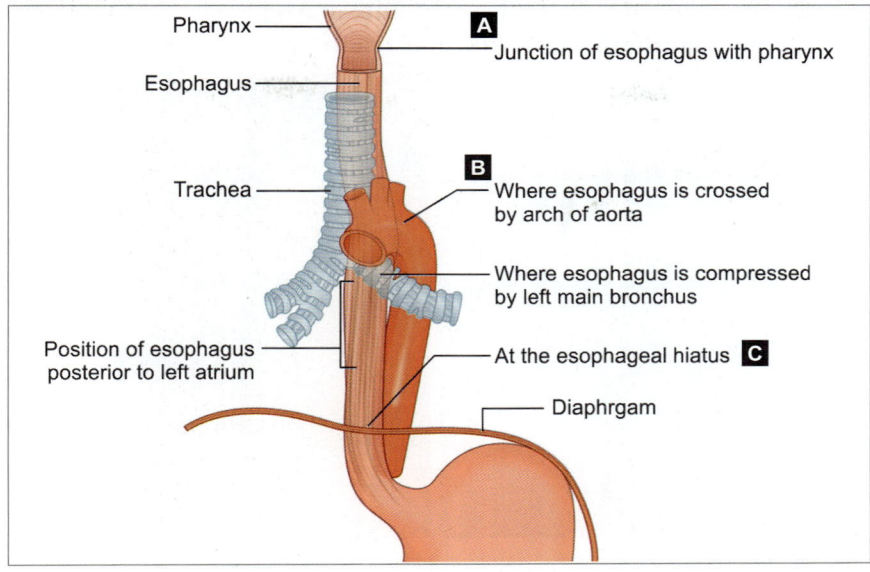

a. What are the levels of the three constrictions of the esophagus shown as A, B and C in the diagram above?
b. What is the length of the esophagus in an adult?
c. What are the three phases in the physiology of swallowing?

Q11. The diagram below shows the major features of a syndrome:

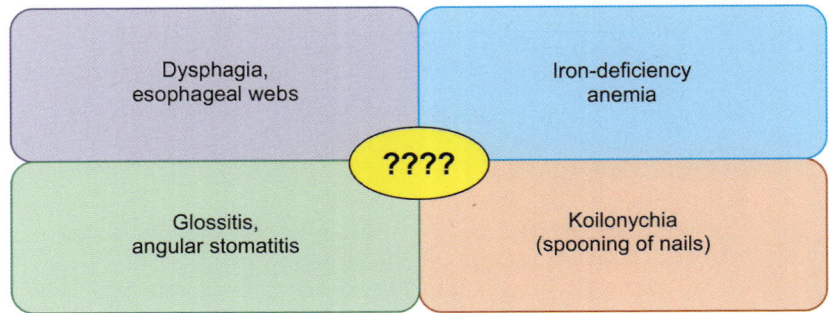

a. What is the syndrome being asked about in the photo?
b. How will you treat this condition?
c. What carcinoma can this condition lead to?

Q12. The images below show a corkscrew and a barium swallow study of a 48-year-old lady with complaints of dysphagia, intermittent odynophagia with substernal chest pain.

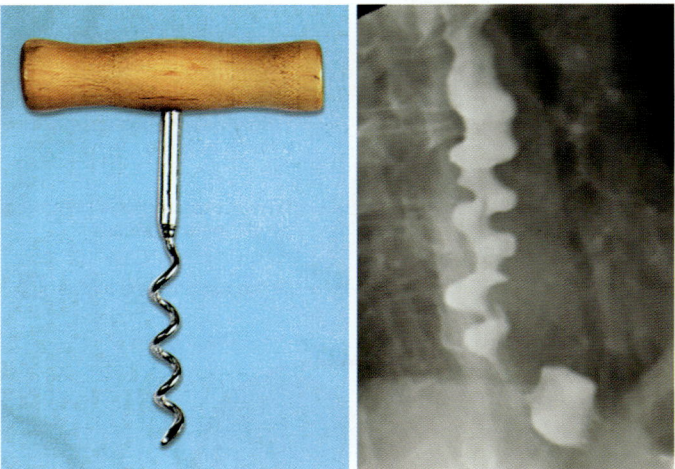

a. Correlate the two images with the patient's complaints to reach to a probable diagnosis.
b. What is the manometry finding in these conditions?
c. What is the treatment?

CHAPTER 14: Pharynx and Esophagus

ANSWERS

Ans 1:
  a. Glossopharyngeal nerve
  b. The glossopharyngeal nerve gives as offshoot—the tympanic nerve, which supplies the tympanic cavity and the tympanic membrane, via which there is referred pain to the ear
  c. i. Tonsillar branch of facial artery (main artery)
     ii. Ascending pharyngeal artery (from external carotid artery)
     iii. Ascending palatine artery (branch of facial artery)

Ans 2:
  a. Grade 3
  b. i. Peritonsillar abscess
     ii. Parapharyngeal abscess
     iii. Tonsillolith/Tonsillar cysts
  c. Infectious mononucleosis—affecting young adults, caused by Epstein-Barr virus (EBV)
  d. Palatoplasty—done in obstructive sleep apnea

Ans 3:
  a. Nasopharynx
  b. i. Fossa of Rosenmuller
     ii. Eustachian Tube (ET) opening
  c. Cervical lymphadenopathy due to cervical nodal metastases (seen in 75% patients on first presentation)

Ans 4:
  a. Proliferative growth in the vallecula on both sides.
  b. i. Base of tongue, ii. Tonsil and tonsillar pillars, iii. Soft palate, iv. Posterior pharyngeal wall
  c. Squamous cell carcinoma

Ans 5:
  a. Zenker's diverticulum/Pharyngeal pouch

Killian triangle	Killian-Jamieson triangle	Laimer triangle
Region between cricopharyngeal and inferior constrictor muscle	Region between the oblique and transverse fibers of the cricopharyngeal muscle	Region between the cricopharyngeal and most superior esophageal circular muscle

  b. Barium swallow study: Pouch will be visualized on anterior or lateral view
  c. i. External diverticulectomy (Cervical incision – trachea, strap muscles, thyroid gland retracted medially, SCM muscle retracted laterally, omohyoid retracted or divided, diverticulum and cricopharyngeus when identified, cricopharyngeal myotomy performed- diverticulum excised – defect closed with purse-string sutures or staples)
     ii. Endoscopic techniques: Laser technique, electrocautery or ultrasonic scissor technique, staple diverticulotomy
     iii. Dohlman's procedure

Ans 6:
   a. Adenoid facies due to adenoid hypertrophy
   b. Conservative with mometasone topical nasal sprays, anti-histaminies, and nasal decongestant drops. If not relieved, surgical management by adenoidectomy under general anesthesia
   c. Digital X-ray soft tissue lateral neck, neck extended, mouth open (to see nasopharynx)

Ans 7:
   a. Bifid uvula
   b. Submucous cleft palate
   c. In patients with submucous cleft palate, bifid uvula might be the only external sign. In such patients, if adenoidectomy is done, it can lead to velopharyngeal insufficiency. If at all it is to be done, partial adenoidectomy, under endoscopic or direct vision should be done, preserving a buttress of tissue around the lateral margins, in order to preserve the velopharyngeal closure mechanism

Ans 8:
   a. Chronic hypertrophic (granular) pharyngitis
   b. i. Foreign body sensation in the throat
      ii. Pain in the throat/discomfort

Ans 9:
   a. Continuous positive airway pressure (CPAP)—provides pneumatic splint to airway and increase its caliber to keep it open, generally the optimum pressure to open the airway during sleep is usually 5–20 cm H_2O. Compliance is poor in 40% cases
   b. Obstructive sleep apnea (OSA) syndrome
   c. Polysomnography (PSG)—Sleep study
   d. Drug induced sleep endoscopy (DISE)

Ans 10:
   a. A–C6, B–T4, C–T10
   b. 25 cm
   c. 3 phases: 1. Oral/Buccal phase; 2. Pharyngeal phase; 3. Esophageal phase

Ans 11:
   a. Plummer-Vinson syndrome (or Paterson-Brown Kelly syndrome)
   b. Correction of anemia (oral/parenteral), dilatation of the webbed areas in esophagus
   c. 10% of cases go on to develop postcricoid carcinoma

Ans 12:
   a. Diffuse esophageal spasm—corksrew type of appearance of esophagus on barium swallow study
   b. Treatment: Dilatation of the lower esophagus, severe case may require – myotomy of esophagus from the arch of aorta to lower sphincter
   c. Manometry shows normal relaxation of the sphincters

CHAPTER 15

Larynx and Trachea

Q1. A 64-year-old male patient presented with hoarseness. A fiberoptic laryngoscopy (FOL) was done for the patient.

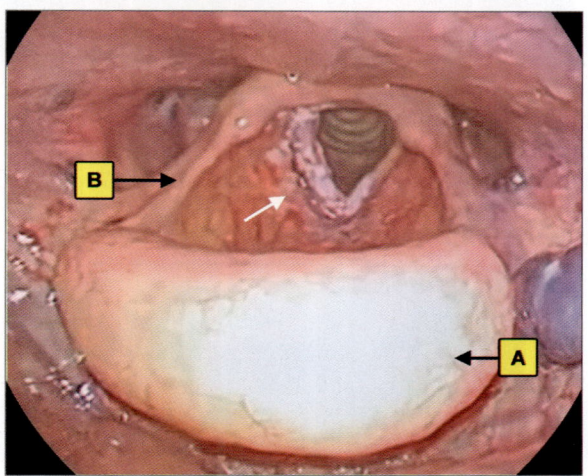

a. What is the diagnosis from the picture above?
b. What is the structure marked as 'A' above?
c. What is the structure marked as 'B' above?
d. What degree endoscopes can be used to perform this procedure–0°/30°/45°/70°/90° rigid endoscopes?

Q2. Observe the photo and answer:

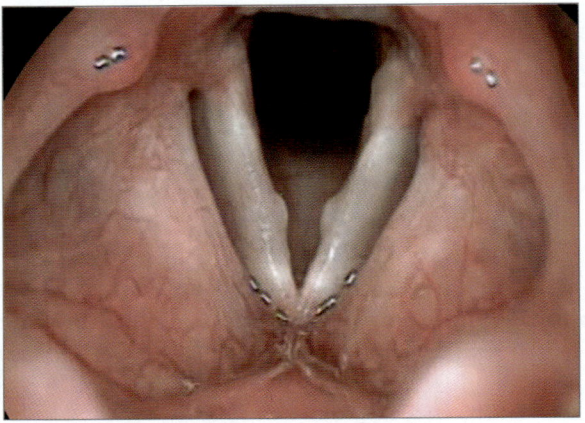

a. What is the pathology shown in the picture?
b. What is the most common cause?
c. What advice will you give to this patient?

Q3. Observe the following photograph:

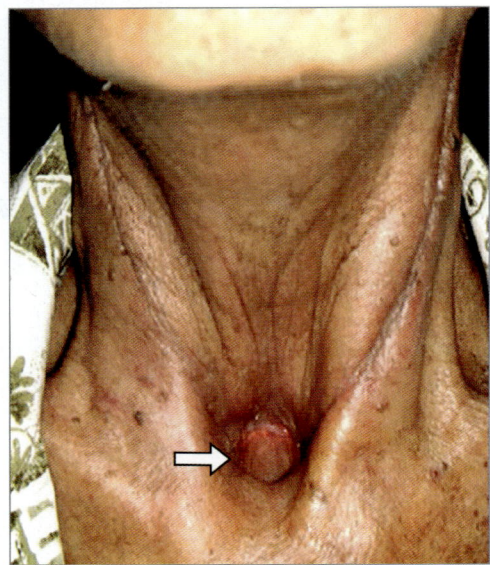

a. What is the opening seen in the picture?
b. What is its indication?

Q4. The following image shows the sagittal section of the larynx:

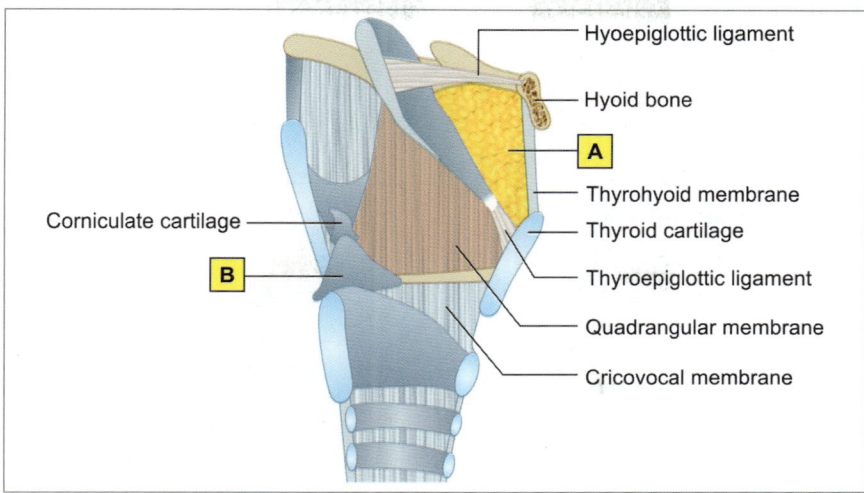

a. Label the structure marked 'B' in the diagram above.
b. What is the space marked by 'A' in the diagram above and what does it contain?
c. What is the applied importance of the space marked as 'A', if involved by laryngeal cancer?

SECTION 3: Throat

Q5. The diagram below shows the coronal section of the larynx:

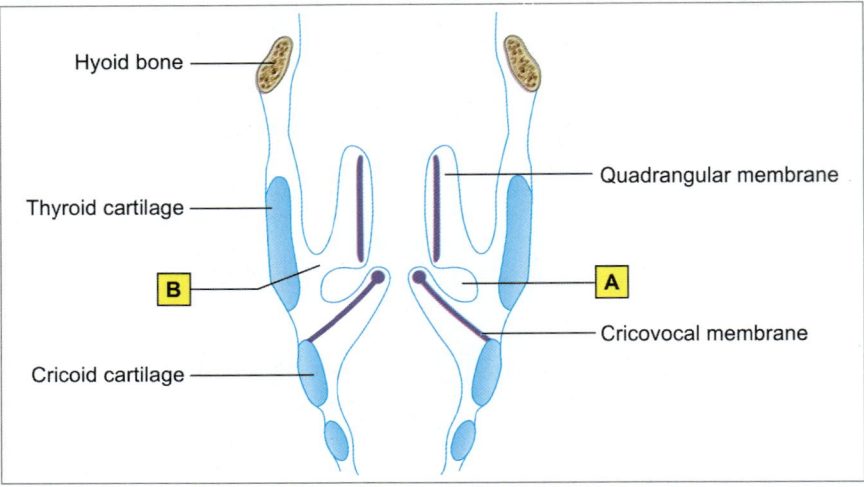

a. What is the structure marked by 'A' in the diagram above?
b. What is the pathological entity that part 'A' can give rise to when abnormally enlarged?
c. What is the area marked by 'B' in the diagram above?
d. What is the applied importance of the area marked by 'B'?
e. Which structure in the above diagram is forming the:
   i. false vocal cord?
   ii. true vocal cord?

Q6. The following diagram shows the intrinsic muscles of the larynx in action:

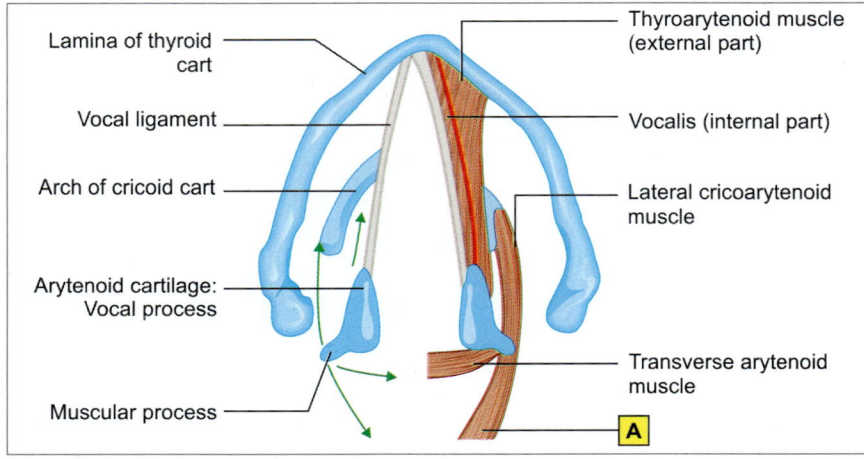

a. What is the muscle marked by 'A'?
b. What is its function?
c. What is the nerve supply of that muscle?
d. Name the two tensors of the vocal cord.

Q7. The following fiberoptic laryngoscopy picture shows a congenital lesion of the larynx in a neonate:

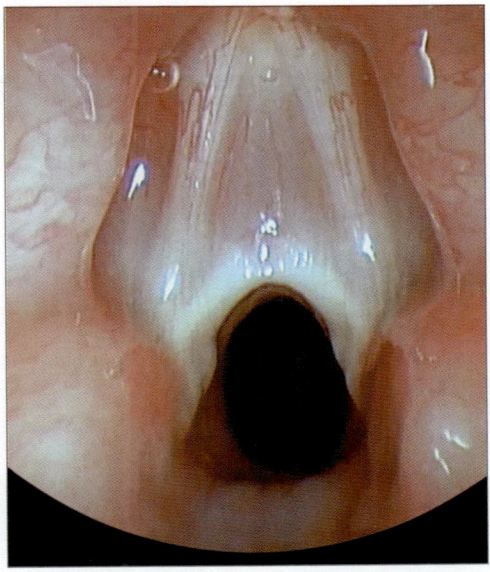

   a. What is the diagnosis?
   b. What will be the presenting features?
   c. What treatment can be given to the baby?

Q8. The following diagram shows the position of the vocal cords in various conditions:

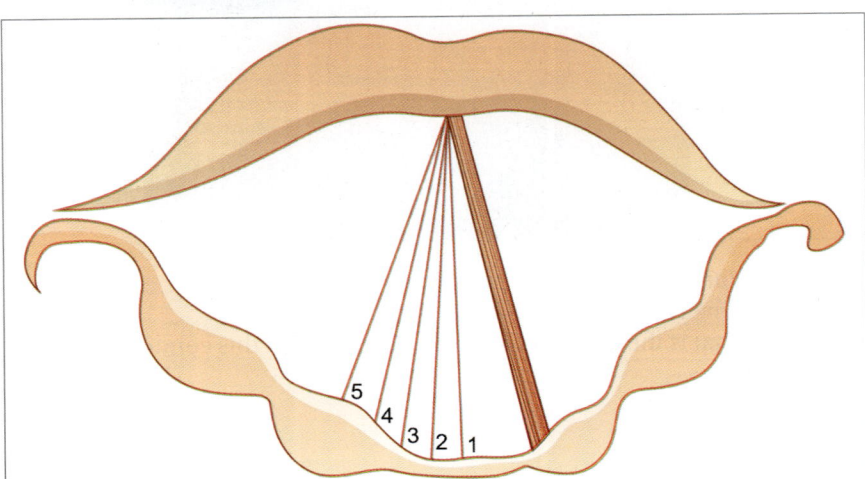

   a. What are the various positions of the cords shown in the diagram from 1–5 and mention the distance of each from the midline?
   b. Which is the position adopted by the cords in paralysis of both recurrent and superior laryngeal nerves?
   c. Which is the position adopted by the cords in quiet respiration?

Q9. The following shows the fiberoptic rigid laryngoscopy (FOL) photograph of an 8-year-old girl who presented with stridor and was managed with definitive surgery after emergency airway management:

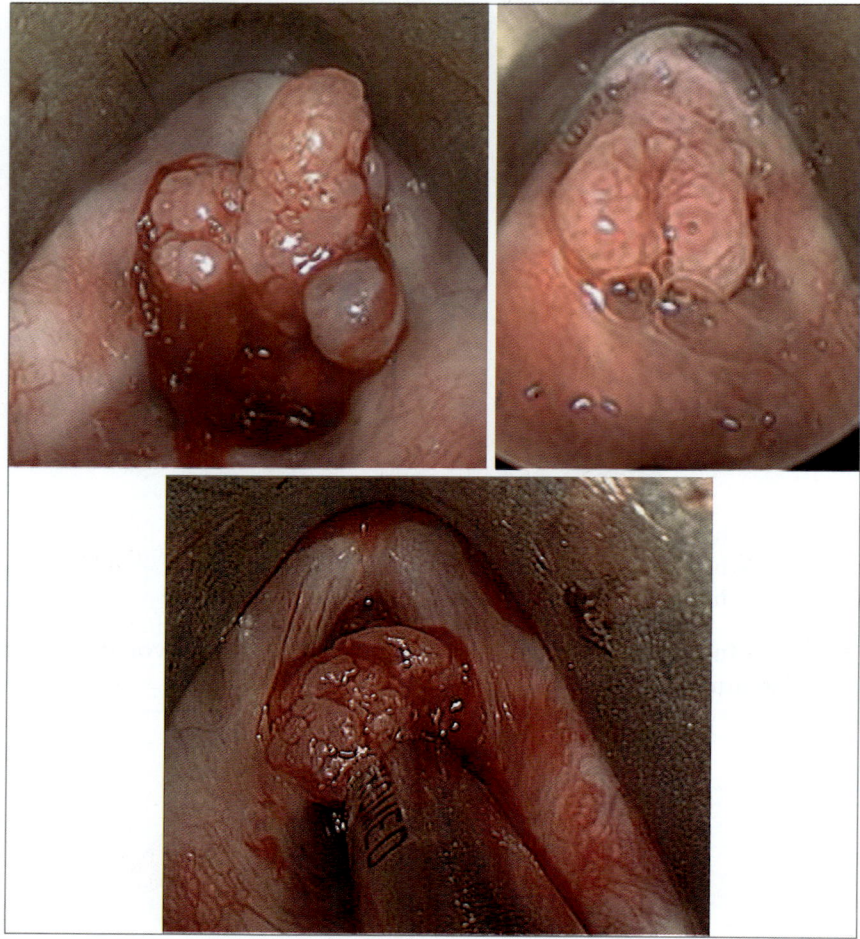

a. What is the diagnosis in this case?
b. What is the causative organism?
c. What is the definitive surgical treatment for this condition?

Q10. The following image shows the use of a device for voice rehabilitation after surgery done in a patient with advanced laryngeal cancer:

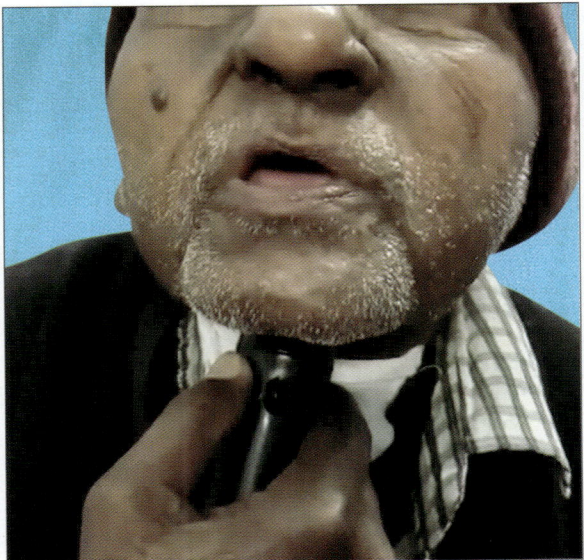

a. What is the surgery that has been performed on this patient?
b. What is the name of the device being used?
c. What is the preferred treatment modality for early laryngeal cancers?

Q11. The following is the fiberoptic laryngoscopy (FOL) image of a 32-year-old lady with hoarseness:

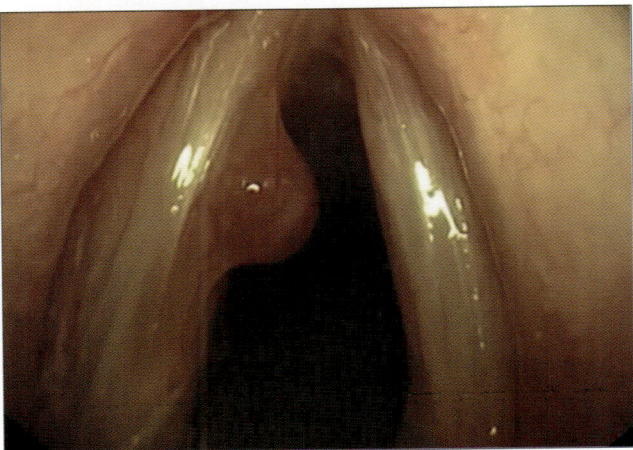

a. What is the diagnosis?
b. What is the treatment?
c. What precaution must the patient follow in the immediate post-operative period?

Q12. The following images are of a 22-year-old boy, presenting with stridor. He had a history of road traffic accident 2 months ago, followed by prolonged intubation for 1 month, and gradual development of respiratory distress after discharge from ICU.

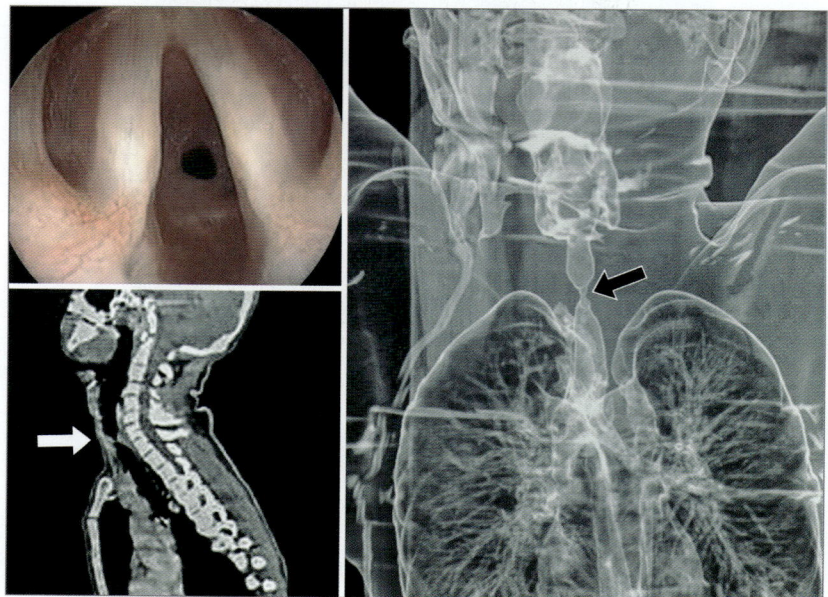

a. What is the diagnosis from the clinical scenario above?
b. What is the grading system used for this condition?
c. What is the emergency management to be done in this patient?

Q13. The following image shows a procedure being performed on a patient:

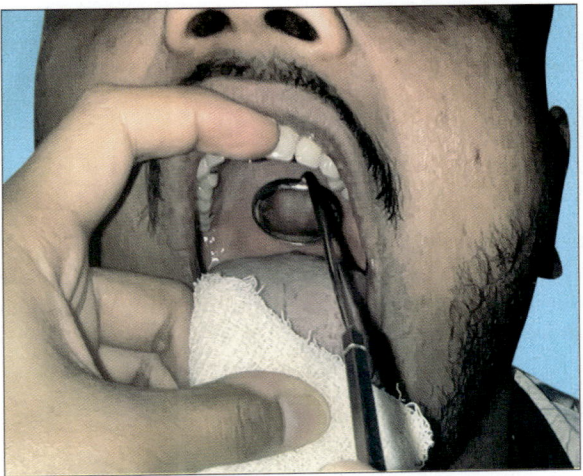

a. What is the procedure being performed?
b. Draw a labelled diagram of the structures seen in this procedure.
c. What is the instrument being used called?
d. How is it prepared before performing the test?

SECTION 3: Throat

ANSWERS

Ans 1:
  a. Glottic growth—Ulceroproliferative growth over right true vocal cord, anterior part of left true vocal cord
  b. Epiglottis
  c. Ary-epiglottic fold (AEF)
  d. 70°/90° rigid endoscopes

Ans 2:
  a. Vocal cord nodule
  b. Vocal abuse: Generally in teachers, professional voice users
  c. Conservative management: with maintaining vocal hygiene, proton-pump inhibitor drugs, steam inhalation

Ans 3:
  a. Permanent stoma post total laryngectomy
  b. Carcinoma larynx

Ans 4:
  a. 'B'—Arytenoid cartilage
  b. 'A'—Pre-epiglottic space of Boyer; contains—fat, loose areolar tissue and some lymphatics
  c. If pre-epiglottic space is involved by laryngeal cancer (T3 disease), radiotherapy cannot be given as the primary modality of definitive therapy, as the area is relatively radioresistant (due to sparse blood supply). Hence surgery has to be contemplated

Ans 5:
  a. 'A'—Ventricle
  b. Laryngocele
  c. 'B'—Paraglottic space; contains—thyroarytenoid muscle
  d. If paraglottic space is involved by laryngeal cancer (T3 disease), thyro-arytenoid muscle gets involved—leading to fixation of the vocal cords
  e. i. Lower free edge of the quadrangular membrane
     ii. Upper free edge of the cricovocal membrane

Ans 6:
  a. Posterior crico-arytenoid muscle
  b. Only abductor of the vocal cords—"safety muscle of larynx"
  c. Recurrent laryngeal nerve (RLN)
  d. i. Cricothyroid muscle
     ii. Vocalis (internal part of thyroarytenoid muscle)

Ans 7:
  a. Laryngeal web
  b. Airway obstruction, weak cry or aphonia
  c. Thin webs: Cut by cold steel instruments or CO_2 laser; thick webs might require excision via laryngofissure and placement of laryngeal keel with subsequent dilatations

Ans 8:
   a. Position of the vocal cords:

Position	Distance from midline	Situation in healthy condition	Situation in disease
1- Median	0 mm	Phonation	RLN paralysis
2- Paramedian	1.5 mm	Strong whisper	RLN paralysis
3- Intermediate (cadaveric)	3.5 mm	-	Paralysis of both recurrent and superior laryngeal nerve
4- Slight abduction	7 mm	Quiet respiration	Paralysis of adductors
5- Full abduction	9.5 mm	Deep inspiration	-

   b. Intermediate (cadaveric) position: This is the neutral position of the crico-arytenoid joint, from which abduction and adduction take place
   c. Slight abduction (7 mm from midline)

Ans 9:
   a. Juvenile onset recurrent respiratory papillomatosis (JORRP)
   b. Human papilloma virus (HPV)—6 and 11
   c. Micro laryngeal surgery (MLS)—removal of the polyps using cold steel, microdebrider or CO_2 laser avoiding injury to the underlying vocal ligament

Ans 10:
   a. Total laryngectomy
   b. Electrolarynx—battery operated, portable device
   c. Radiotherapy

Ans 11:
   a. Right true vocal cord cyst
   b. Micro laryngeal surgery (MLS)—excision of cyst
   c. Absolute voice rest

Ans 12:
   a. Subglottic stenosis (Post prolonged intubation)
   b. Cotton-Myer grading
   c. Emergency tracheostomy to be done, to bypass the stenotic part of the airway

Ans 13:
    a. Indirect laryngoscopy
    b. Labelled diagram of structures seen in indirect laryngoscopy:

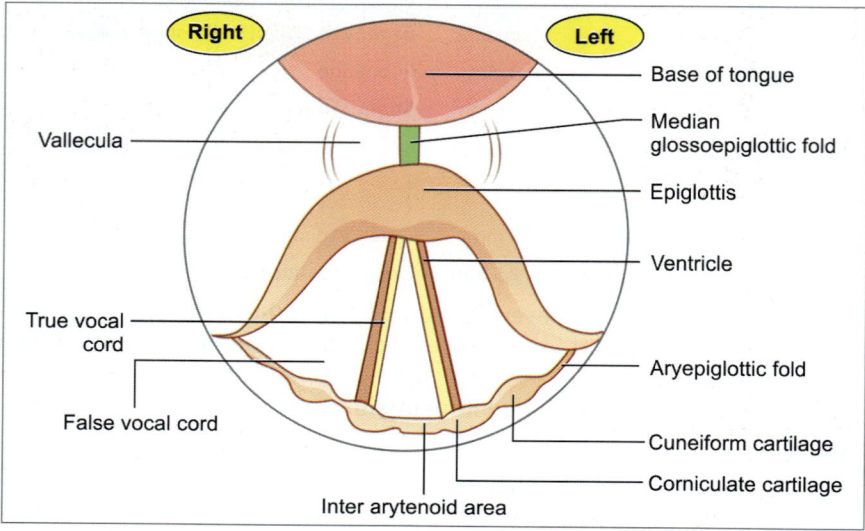

    c. Laryngeal mirror
    d. The laryngeal mirror is warmed and tested on the back of the hand. Alternatively, anti-fogging solution (like Savlon) can be used

NECK

SECTION 4

SECTION OUTLINE

16. Neck Proper
17. Thyroid and Parathyroid Glands

CHAPTER 16

Neck Proper

Q1. The following diagram shows the various lymph node levels in the neck:

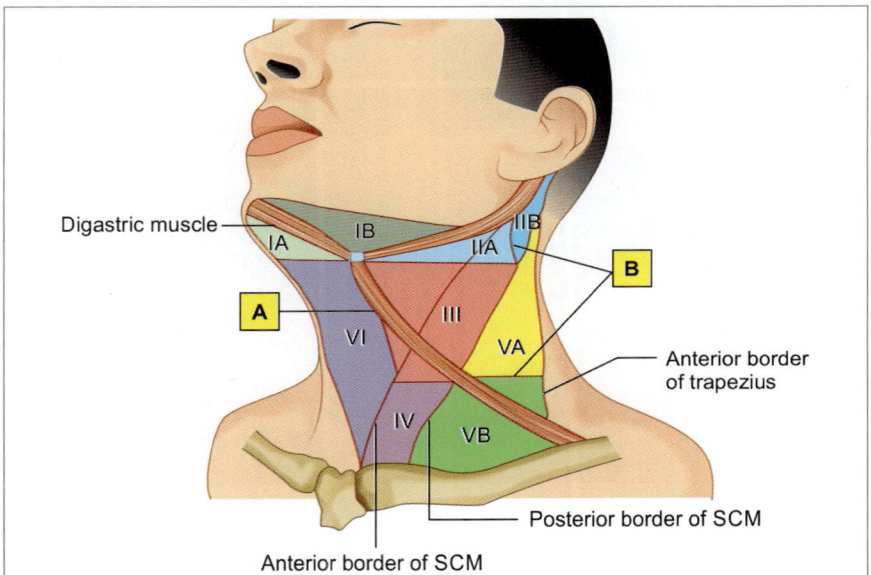

a. What is the name of the muscle marked as 'A'?
b. What is the name of the structure indicated as 'B'?
   (**HINT!** 'B' is a **nerve**...subdividing level II into IIA and IIB and running across the roof of level V)
c. What are some other names of level VII nodes? (Name 3)
d. Which structure forms the lateral boundaries of the level VII lymph nodes?

Q2. The following images show an examination being done on a patient:

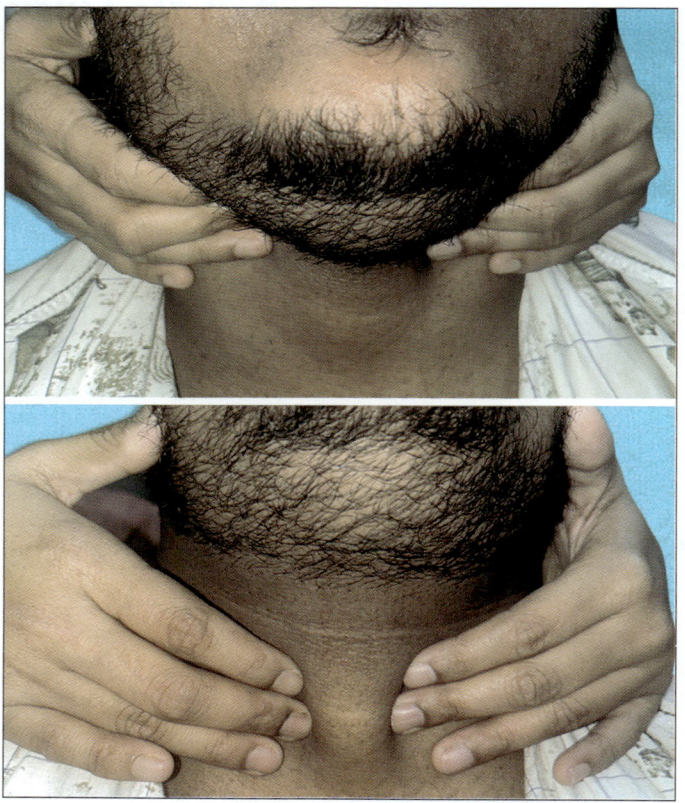

a. What is the examination being done?
b. What is the position of the examiner for this procedure with respect to the patient?
c. What should be the position of the patient's neck?

Q3. The following is a clinical photograph of a 12-year-old boy with a midline neck swelling moving with deglutition and protrusion of tongue:

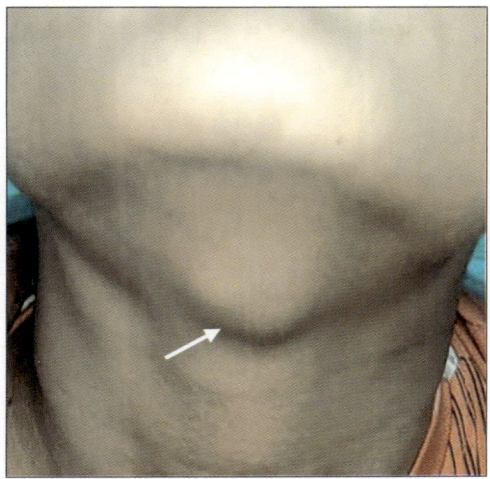

a. What is the probable diagnosis?
b. What are the 2 specific investigations will you order for this boy?
c. What is the treatment of choice?

Q4. The following image is of a 9-year-old boy, having history of caries tooth for the last 2 weeks, developing a rapid painful swelling in the neck:

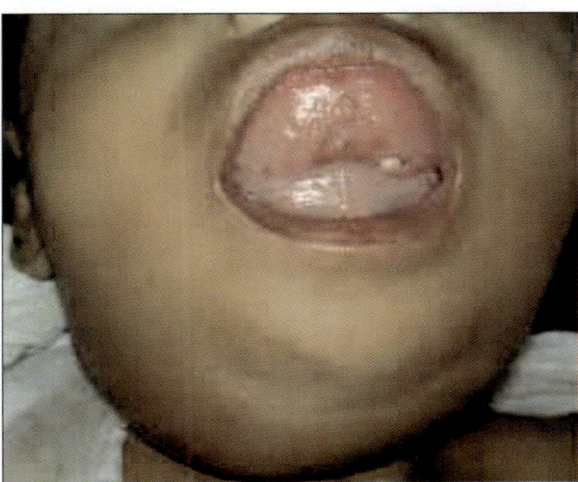

a. What is the diagnosis from the photograph being shown?
b. Relating to the finding in the oral cavity from the image, what is this appearance known as?
c. What is the treatment you will give?
d. Mention 3 complications that can occur.

Q5. The illustration below shows the various types of neck dissections:

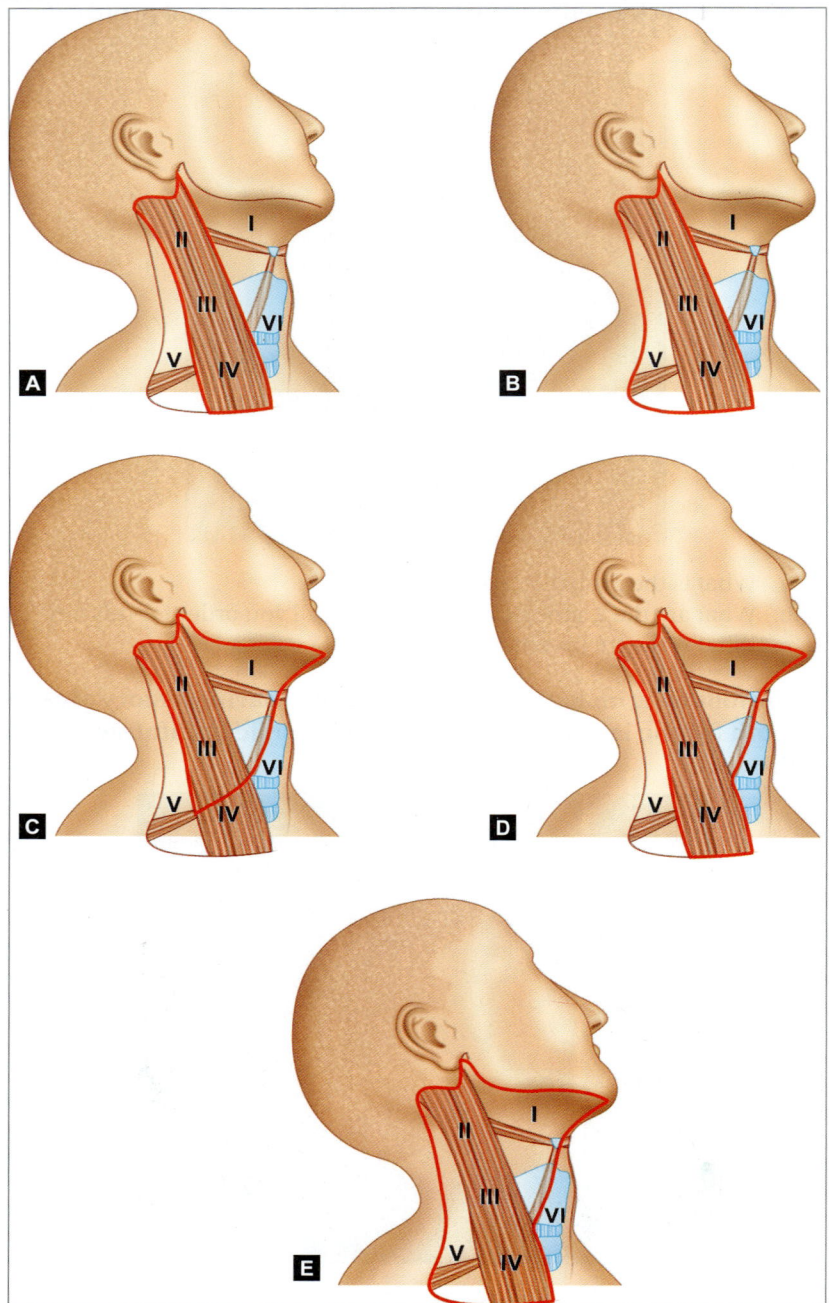

a. Write the names of the various types of neck dissections as shown from A to E in the diagram above.
b. What are the three structures that are preserved in modified radical neck dissection (MRND)?

Q6. The illustrations below show two types of incisions for neck dissection:

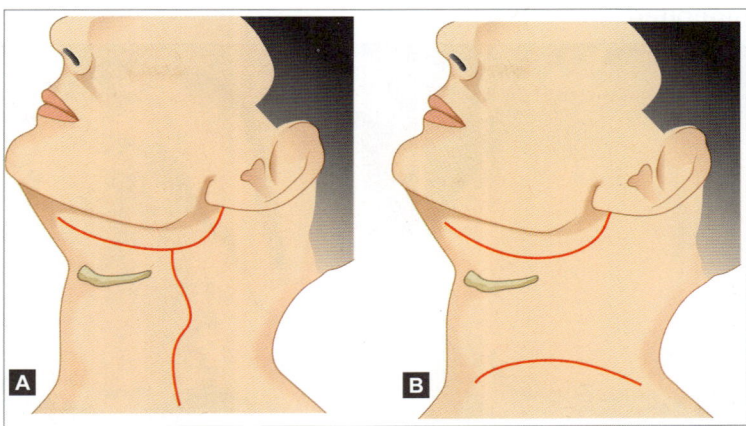

a. What is 'A' and 'B'?
b. What is the incision used generally for total laryngectomy with neck dissection?
c. What is Ho's triangle? What lymph nodes does it have?

Q7. The following is a 36-year-old lady with a swelling on the left side of her neck.

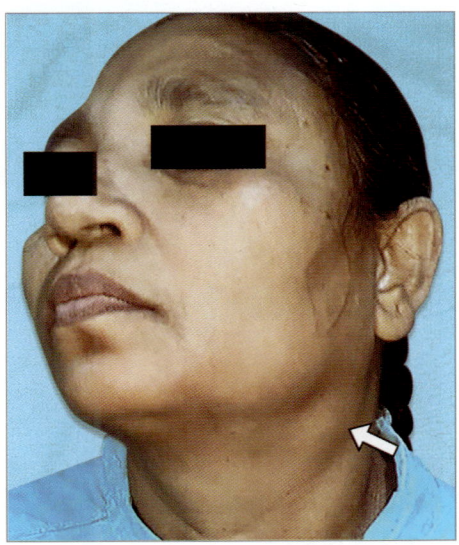

a. Give 3 differential diagnoses of lateral neck swellings.
b. What is the sign seen on MR angiography of a patient with a carotid body tumor, due to splaying of the internal and external carotid arteries?
c. What blood investigations should you order in order to check if a carotid body tumor is of the functional and secreting type?

SECTION 4: Neck

Q8. The following are the photographs of a 43-year-old lady, with a huge, soft, cystic and brightly transilluminant swelling which was operated:

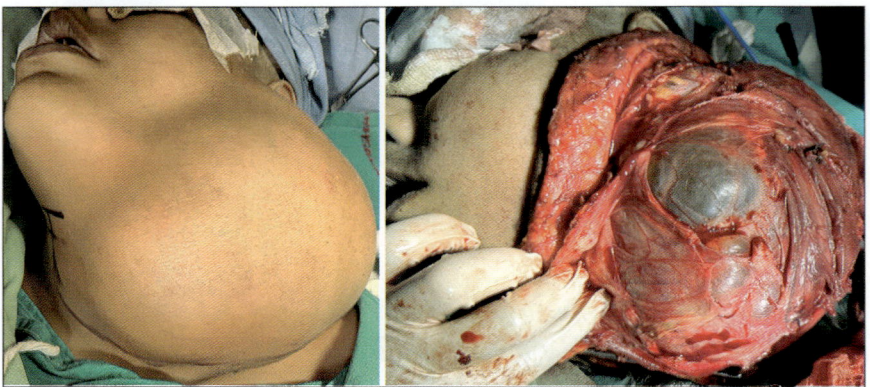

a. What is the most probable diagnosis?
b. What is the danger/emergency related to such swellings?

Q9. The following is the photograph of a 25-year-old male with the complaint of discharging sinuses on both sides of the lower neck:

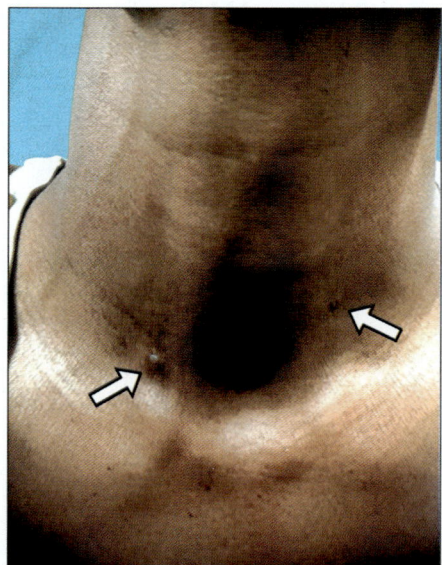

a. What is the diagnosis?
b. What is the most common arch of origin of this clinical entity?
c. What is the treatment for this condition?

CHAPTER 16: Neck Proper

Q10. A 55-year-old man presented to the ENT OPD with the following swelling, progressively increasing since 1 year. It is non-tender and soft.

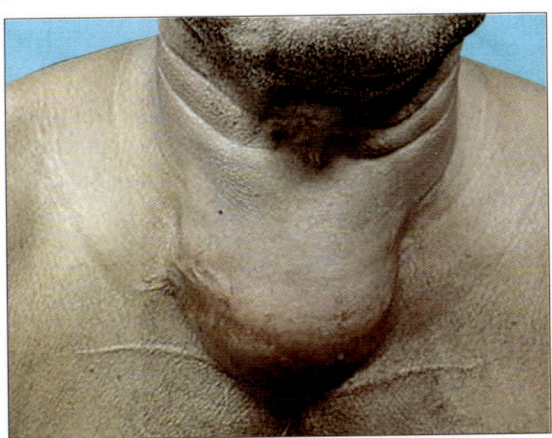

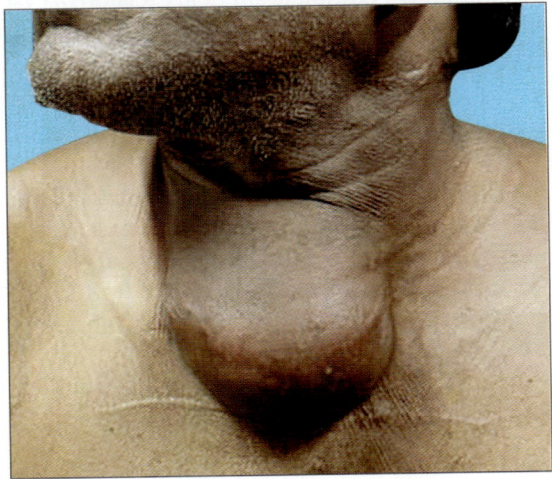

a. What is the first investigation you will order for this patient?
b. Give three differentials for a midline neck swelling.
c. Which branchial arch derivative is thymus?

ANSWERS

Ans 1:
   a. Omohyoid muscle
   b. Spinal accessory nerve (SAN)
   c. Anterior cervical lymph node or central compartment also known as: Paratracheal, delphian (precricoid), perithyroid lymph nodes
   d. Common carotid arteries on either side – form the lateral boundaries

Ans 2:
   a. Examination of the neck
   b. Examiner stands behind the patient
   c. Slightly flexed

Ans 3:
   a. Thyroglossal duct cyst
   b. i. Ultrasonography of the neck and thyroid
       ii. FNAC (fine needle aspiration cytology) from the swelling
   c. Sistrunk operation—complete surgical excision of cyst with its entire tract, including the body of the hyoid bone, core of tongue tissue around the tract up to foramen cecum

Ans 4:
   a. Ludwig's angina
   b. Double tongue appearance
   c. (i) Incision and drainage and sending sample (if present) for culture. Cellulitis is more commonly present than frank abscess, (ii) Systemic antibiotics, (iii) Tracheostomy may be necessary if there is impending airway compromise
   d. Three complications:
       i. Airway obstruction
       ii. Spread of infection to parapharyngeal/retropharyngeal spaces
       iii. Septicemia

Ans 5:
   a. A: Lateral neck dissection
      B: Postero-lateral neck dissection
      C: Supraomohyoid neck dissection (SOND)
      D: Antero-lateral neck dissection
      E: Modified radical neck dissection (MRND)
   b. i. Spinal accessory nerve (cranial nerve XI)
       ii. Internal jugular vein
       iii. Sternocleidomastoid muscle

Ans 6:
   a. A: Schobinger Incision
      B: McFee Incision
   b. Gluck-Sorenson incision
   c. Supraclavicular fossa is Ho's triangle. Contains lymph nodes—Level IV and Level V (lower portions of each)

Ans 7:
- a. Three differential diagnoses:
    i. Jugular lymph nodes (lymphadenopathy)
    ii. Branchial cyst
    iii. Paraganglioma
- b. Lyre's sign—A lyre is a small U-shaped, stringed musical instrument, which was used in ancient Greece

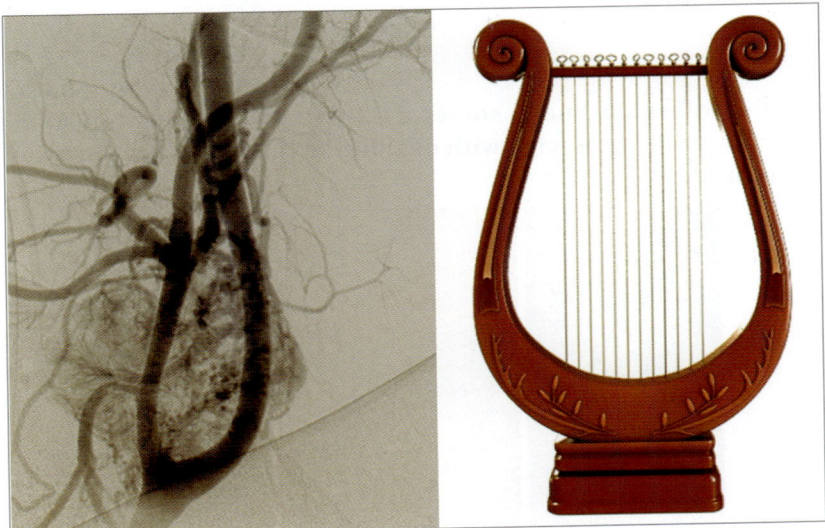

- c. Serum catecholamines, urinary metanephrines and vanillylmandelic acid (VMA)

Ans 8:
- a. Lymphangioma
- b. Involvement of laryngeal/pharyngeal structures due to increase in size/infection—leading to airway compromise – stridor, respiratory difficulty, dysphagia – might need emergency airway management

Ans 9:
- a. Branchial sinus or fistula
- b. Second branchial arch
- c. Complete surgical excision of the tract by step-ladder incisions

Ans 10:
- a. Ultrasonography of neck
- b. (i) Lipoma, (ii) Thyroglossal cyst, (iii) Dermoid cyst
- c. Third arch (third pharyngeal pouch)

Thyroid and Parathyroid Glands

Q1. The following image shows a 33-year-old lady with a midline neck swelling moving with deglutition but not with protrusion of tongue.

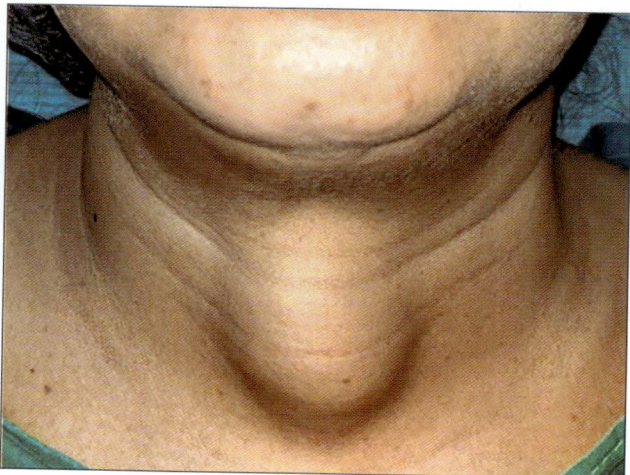

a. What is the first imaging modality you will order for this patient?
b. What is the blood test you should order for this patient?
c. What does TIRADS stand for?
d. What is a positive Pemberton's sign?

Q2. The following image shows a mass at the base of the tongue in a 10 year old male presenting in the ENT OPD, raising the suspicion of a lingual thyroid:

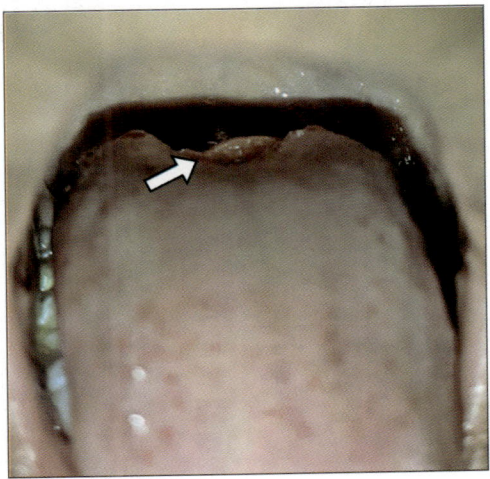

a. What investigation will you order for this patient and why?
b. Give 3 other differentials for this mass.

Q3. The diagram below shows the view as seen from laterally during thyroidectomy:

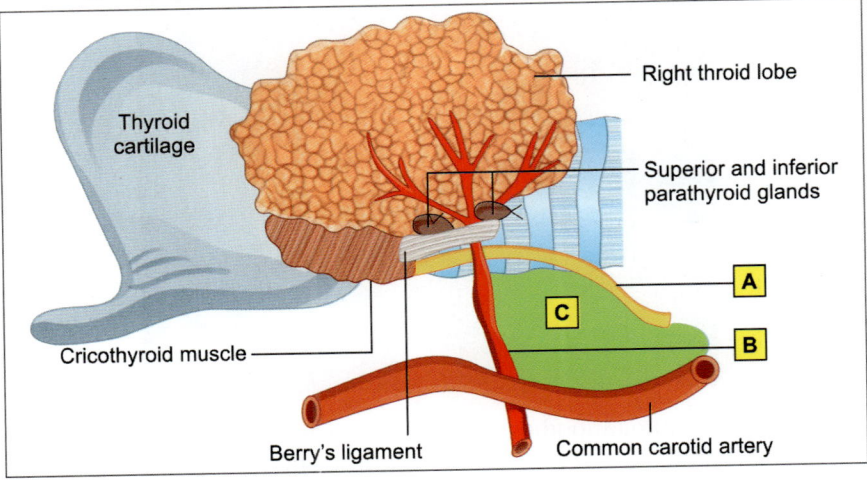

a. What are the structures marked as 'A' and 'B'?
b. What is the green shaded area, marked with 'C' showing?
c. What is the surgical importance of the area 'C'?

Q4. The diagram below shows structures seen during dissection of the upper pole of the thyroid gland:

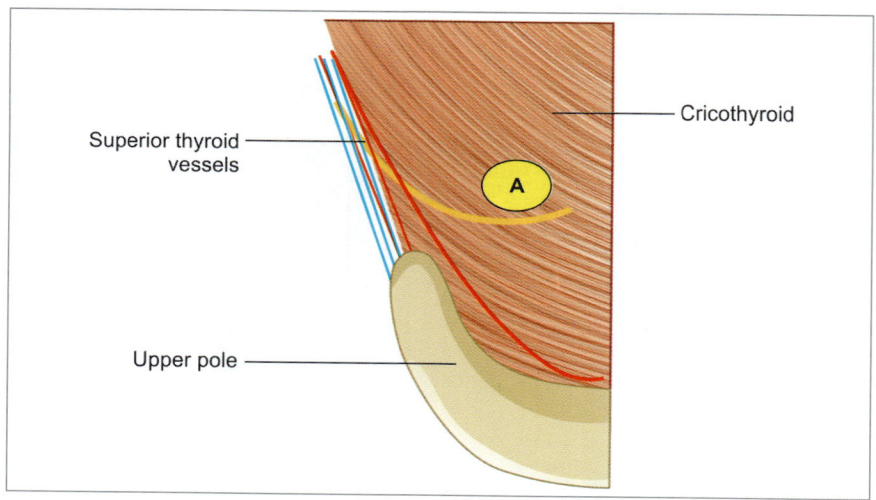

a. What is the name of the triangle shown here?
b. What is the structure marked as 'A'?
c. What structures are forming the floor and roof of this triangle?

Q5. The following image shows a patient with Graves' disease:

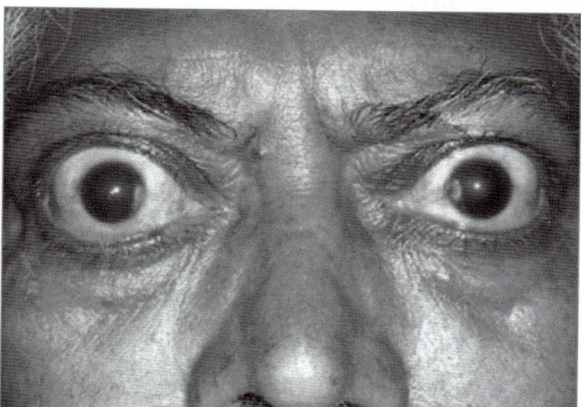

a. Which autoantibodies are seen in Graves' disease?
b. Accumulation of which substance leads to the lesions of the thyroid eye disease?
c. What treatment can you give in early stage of eye disease?

Q6. The following illustration shows the surgical options for management of the thyroid gland:

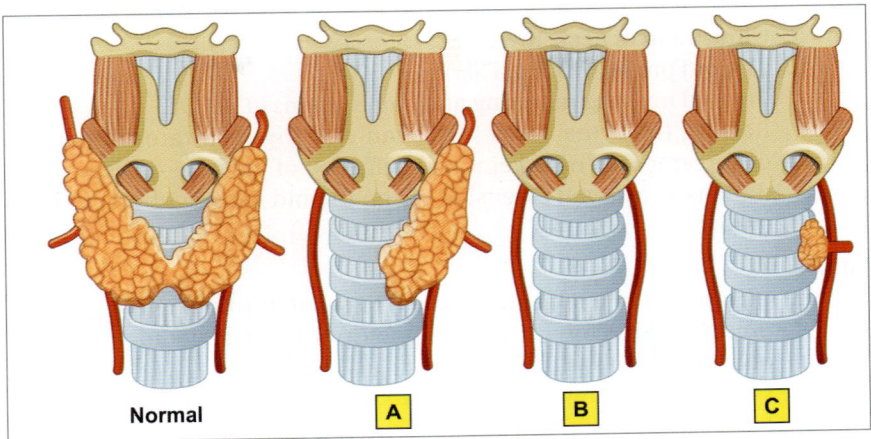

a. Label the types of thyroid surgery shown by 'A', 'B', 'C'.
b. What is completion thyroidectomy?
c. What weight of thyroid tissue is left behind on each side in subtotal thyroidectomy?

ANSWERS

Ans 1:
    a. Ultrasound of neck/thyroid
    b. Thyroid profile (T3, T4, TSH)
    c. Thyroid imaging reporting and data systems (TIRADS)
    d. Raising the arms above the head causing respiratory distress, engorgement of neck veins and suffusion of the face—occurs when there is substernal extension of the thyroid causing thoracic-inlet syndrome

Ans 2:
    a. Ultrasound of neck and thyroid—To see if normal thyroid gland is present or an ectopic thyroid. Sometimes, lingual thyroid may be the only thyroid tissue that is present
    b. Differentials: Lymphoma, squamous cell carcinoma, lingual tonsil

Ans 3:
    a. 'A'—Recurrent laryngeal nerve (RLN)
       'B'—Inferior thyroid artery (ITA)
    b. 'C'—Beahr's triangle (3 sides formed by RLN, ITA, CCA)
    c. Surgical importance: Useful for identification of the recurrent laryngeal nerve (RLN) during thyroid surgery, as it forms the medial boundary

Ans 4:
    a. Joll's triangle
    b. External branch of the superior laryngeal nerve (EBSLN)
    c. Floor: Cricothyroid muscle (shown in picture)

Ans 5:
    a. Autoantibodies to TSH receptors
    b. Accumulation of glycosaminoglycans secreted by the retroorbital fibroblasts - cause engorgement of extraocular muscles and orbital fat and increase the volume of orbital contents
    c. High dose systemic corticosteroids - can be used for the management of early Grave's ophthalmopathy

Ans 6:
    a. A—Hemithyroidectomy
       B—Total thyroidectomy
       C—Near-total thyroidectomy
    b. Completion thyroidectomy—refers to removal of the remaining thyroid gland at a second stage surgery, after an ominous histology is received in the first surgery
    c. 3 grams

SECTION 5

INSTRUMENTS

SECTION OUTLINE

18. OPD Instruments
19. OT Instruments

CHAPTER 18

OPD Instruments

GENERAL

Q1.

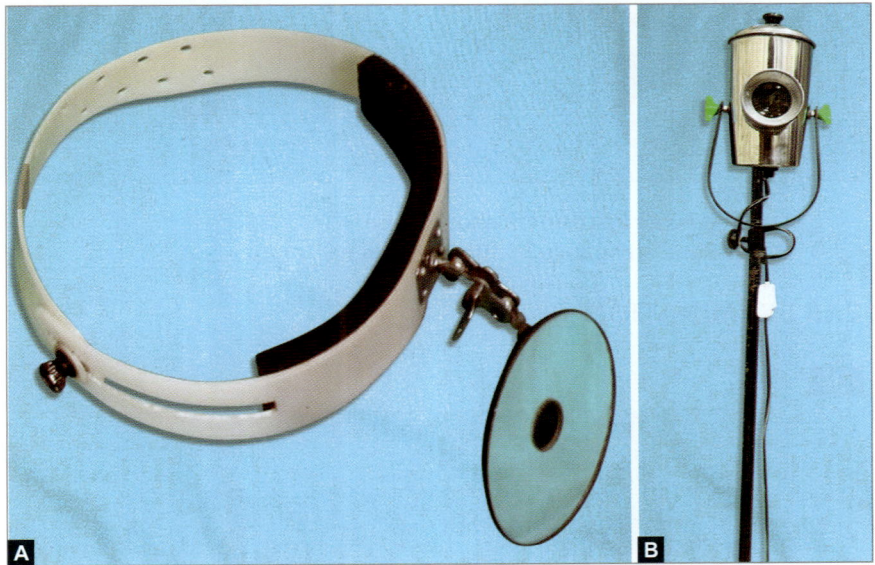

a. Identify these instruments—'A' and 'B'.
b. What is the focal length of this instrument 'A'?
c. What is the use of these instruments?
d. What is the type of mirror used in 'A'—concave or convex?

SECTION 5: Instruments

Q2.

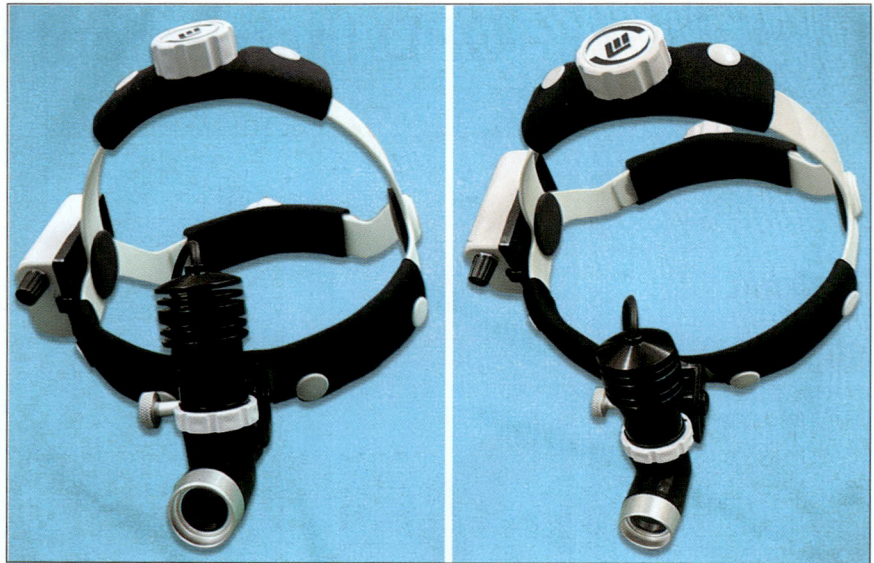

a. What is the instrument shown here?
b. Give one advantage of this instrument.

EAR EXAMINATION

Q1.

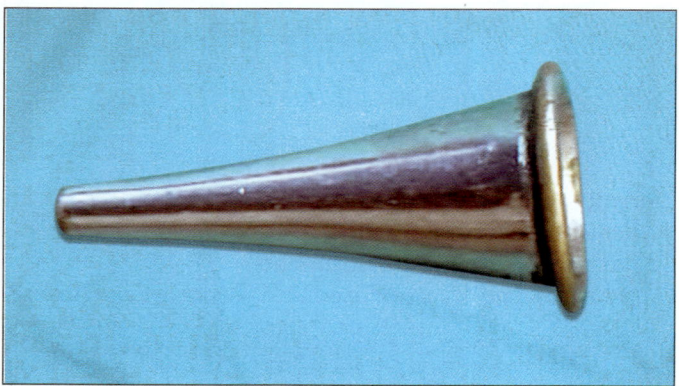

a. Identify the instrument.
b. Write down the uses of this instrument?

CHAPTER 18: OPD Instruments 137

Q2.

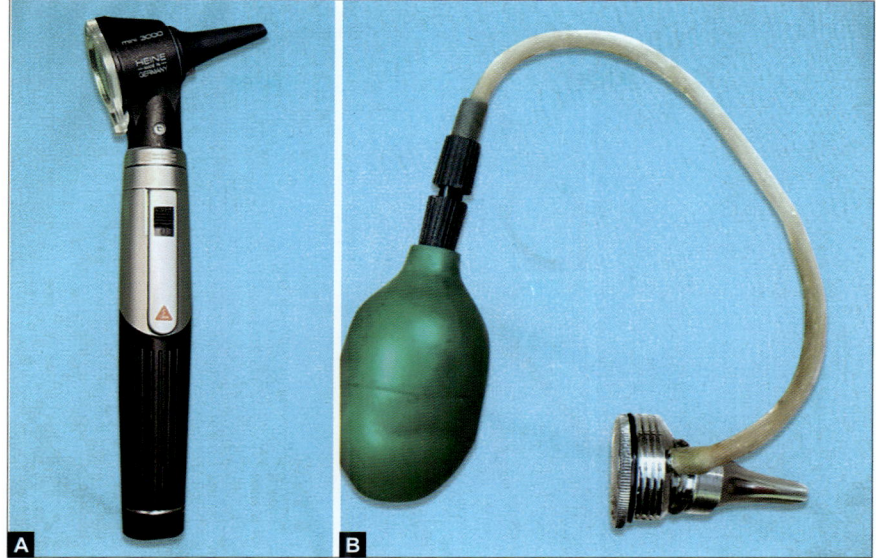

a. Identify the 2 instruments shown.
b. What are its uses?

Q3.

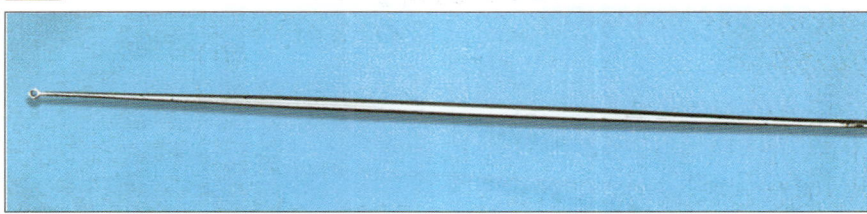

a. Identify the instrument.
b. What are its uses.

Q4. Observe the two instruments below:

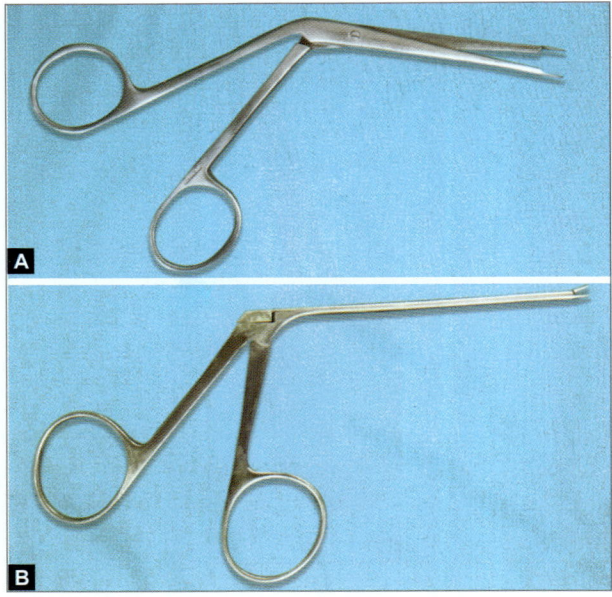

a. What are the two instruments being shown in A and B?
b. Give two uses of the instrument shown in A.

NASAL EXAMINATION

Q1.

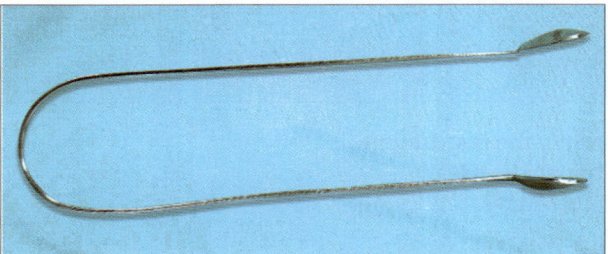

a. Identify this instrument.
b. What is its use?

Q2.

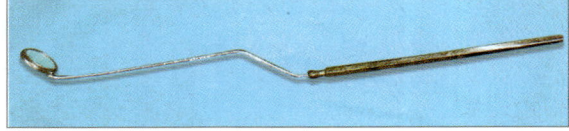

a. Identify this instrument.
b. What is its use?

Q3.

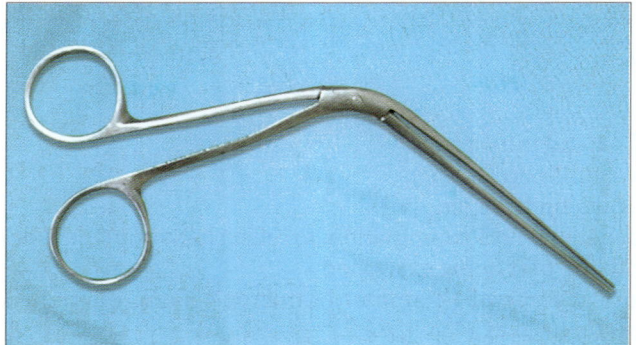

a. Identify this instrument.
b. What is its use?

THROAT EXAMINATION

Q1.

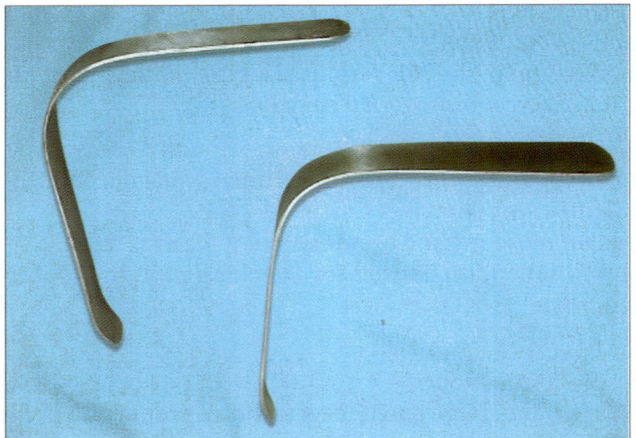

a. Identify this instrument.
b. What is its use?

Q2.

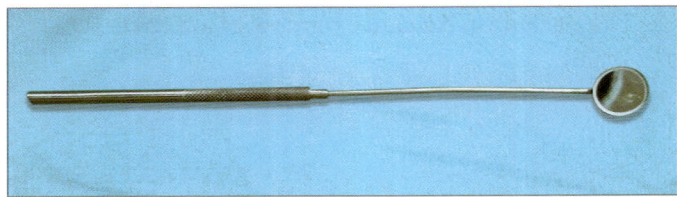

a. Identify this instrument.
b. What are the structures seen by this instrument?

SECTION 5: Instruments

ANSWERS

GENERAL

Ans 1:
- a. 'A'—Head mirror
  'B'—Bull's eye lamp
- b. Focal length: 25 cm
- c. For general ENT examination, to reflect light from the Bull's eye lamp onto the part being examined
- d. Concave mirror (diameter of mirror – 9 cm, diameter of central aperture –2 cm)

Ans 2:
- a. Head light
- b. It allows for bedside examination, as it is portable and battery-operated

EAR EXAMINATION

Ans 1:
- a. Aural speculum
- b. Examination of the ear, various sizes are available for inserting into various sizes of the external ear canal

Ans 2:
- a. A: Otoscope: (has convex lens which gives magnification of two times)
  B: Siegel's speculum
- b. Used for otoscopy and examination of the ear
  Siegel's speculum is used for checking mobility of the tympanic membrane

Ans 3:
- a. Jobson-Horne probe
- b. It has two ends. One end is used to form a cotton bud to clean the ear of discharge and the other end (with ring curette) is used to remove the wax

Ans 4:
- a. A: Hartman's forceps
  B: Crocodile forceps
- b. Used for packing in ear canal, removal of foreign body

NASAL EXAMINATION

Ans 1:
   a. Thudichum's nasal speculum
   b. Performing anterior rhinoscopy

Ans 2:
   a. Postnasal mirror
   b. For performing posterior rhinoscopy, examine the nasopharynx and posterior part of nasal cavity

Ans 3:
   a. Tilley's dressing forceps
   b. Nasal packing, foreign body removal

THROAT EXAMINATION

Ans 1:
   a. Lack's tongue depressor
   b. Examination of the oral cavity, oropharynx, for posterior rhinoscopy, for oral cavity procedures like injecting steroids, biopsy, excision of cyst, etc.

Ans 2:
   a. Laryngeal mirror
   b. Various sizes from 6–30 mm diameter are available for examination of the laryngopharynx

CHAPTER 19

OT Instruments

GENERAL

Q1.

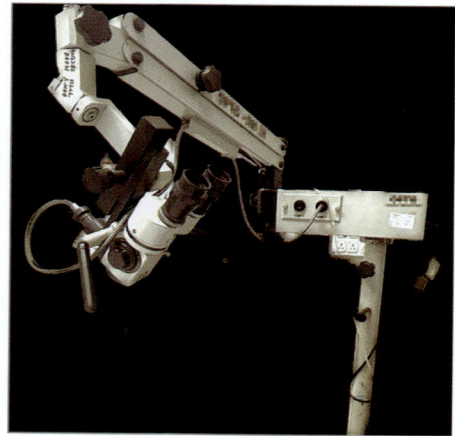

a. What is the instrument shown in the image?
b. What is the range of magnification provided by it?
c. What objective lens is used for ear/ nose/ larynx?

Q2.

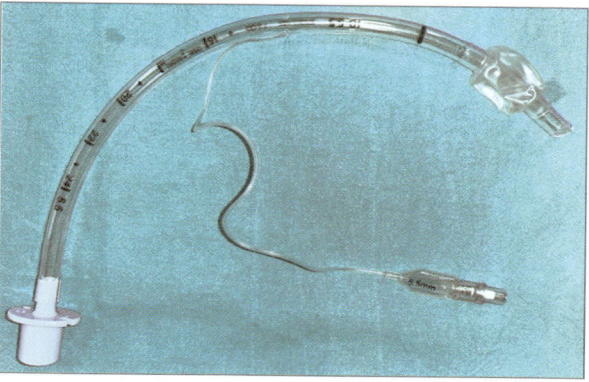

a. Identify this tube.
b. What is it used for?

Q3.

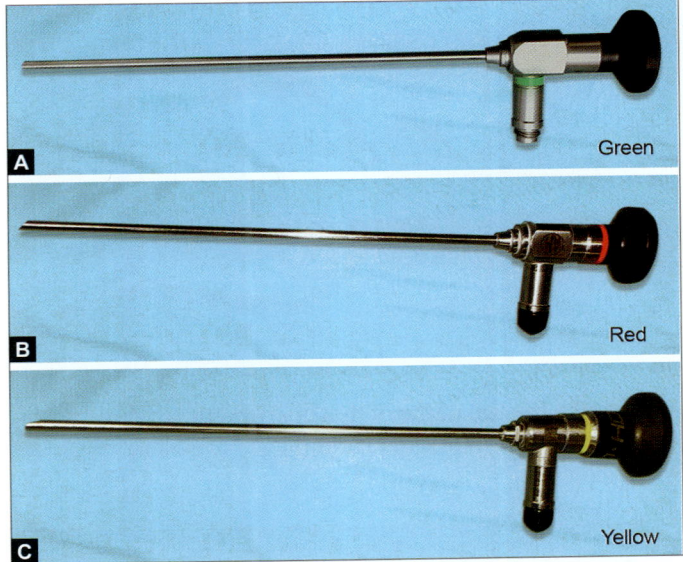

A — Green
B — Red
C — Yellow

a. What are the angulations of the various nasal endoscopes shown in the images above?
b. What is the diameter of these endoscopes?

EAR SURGERY

Q1.

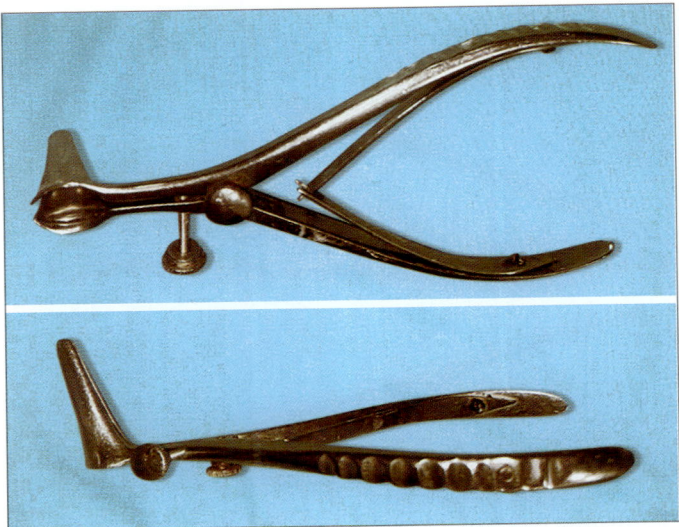

a. Identify this instrument.
b. What is its use?

Q2.

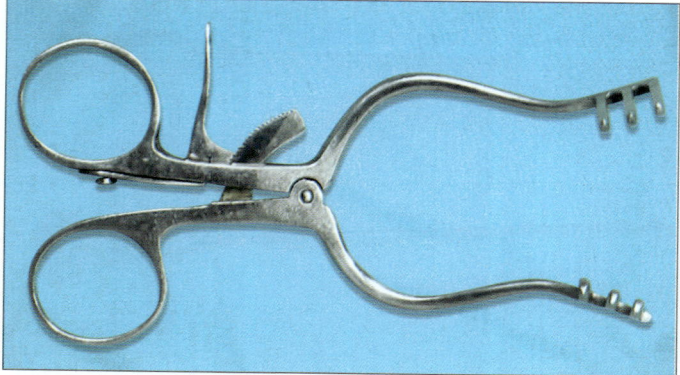

a. Write down the full name of this instrument.
b. Mention one use of this instrument.

Q3.

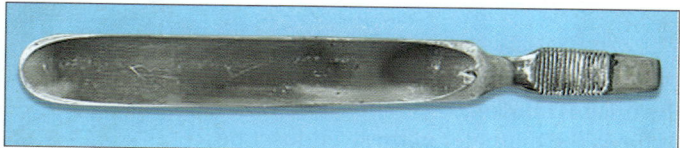

a. Identify this instrument.
b. What is its use?

Q4. The following image shows burrs used in ENT:

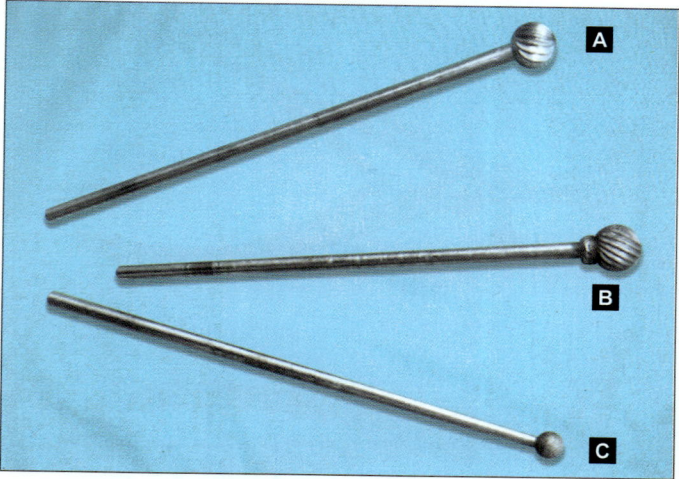

a. Identify the types of the burrs A, B, and C.
b. What surgery can it be used in?

CHAPTER 19: OT Instruments   145

NASAL SURGERY

Q1.

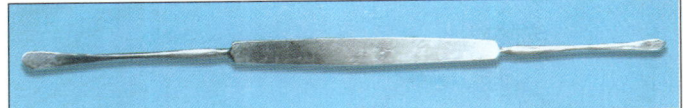

    a. What is the instrument shown here?
    b. What are its uses.

Q2.

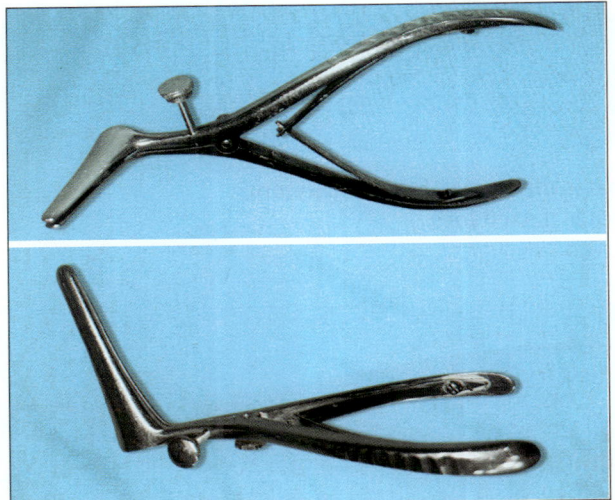

    a. What is the name of this instrument?
    b. What are its uses.

Q3.

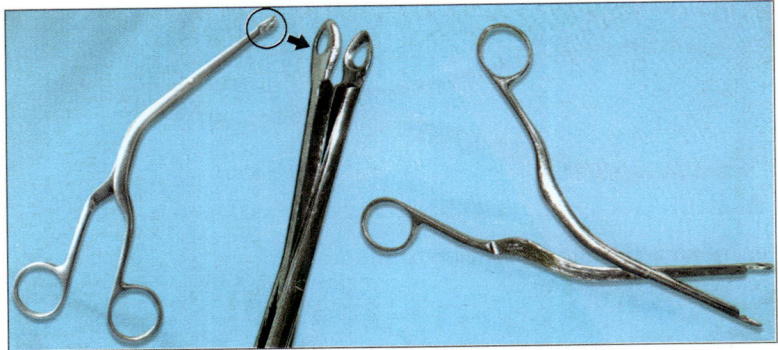

    a. What is the name of this instrument?
    b. What are its uses.
    c. What is the joint present in this instrument?

Q4.

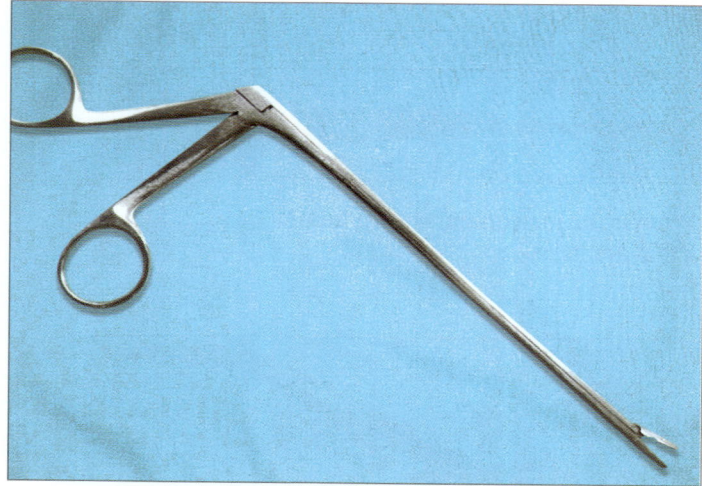

a. What is the name of the instrument?
b. What is it used for?

Q5.

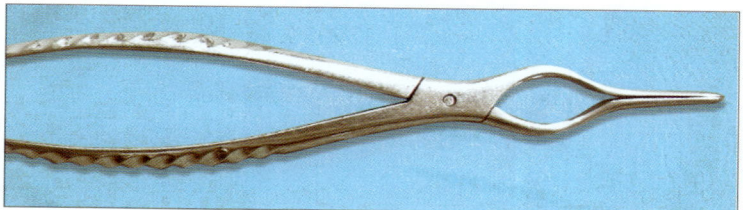

a. What is the name of the instrument?
b. What is it used for?

Q6.

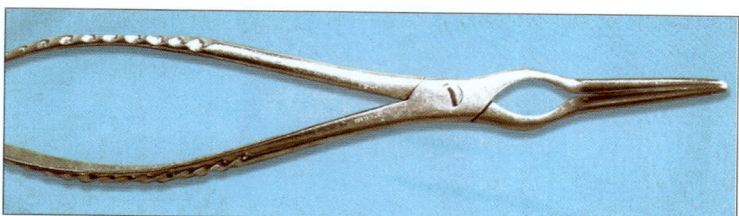

a. What is the name of the instrument?
b. What is it used for?

THROAT/OROPHARYNGEAL SURGERY

Q1.

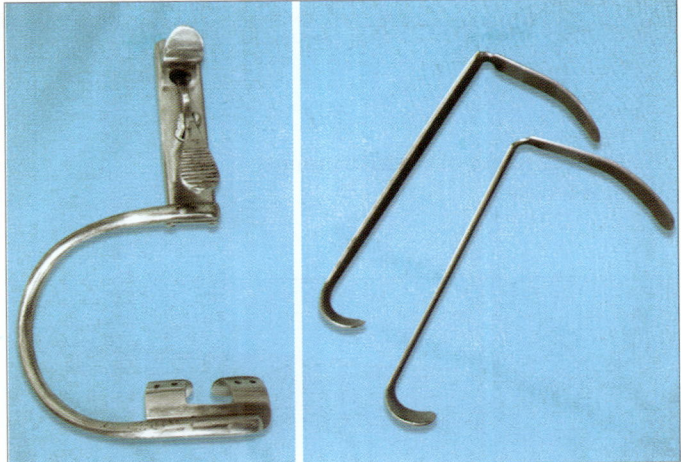

    a. What is the name of the instrument?
    b. What surgery is it used in?

Q2.

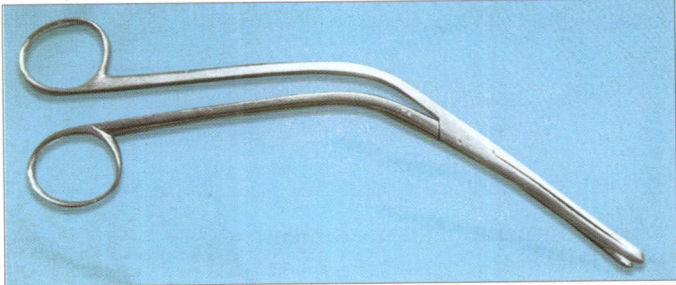

    a. What is the name of the instrument?
    b. What surgery is it used in?

Q3.

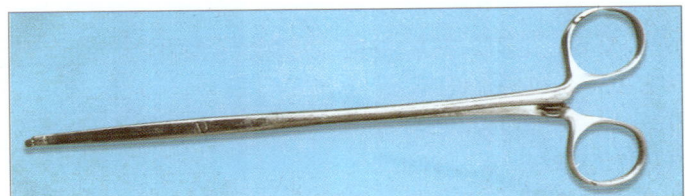

    a. What is the name of the instrument?
    b. What is its use?

SECTION 5: Instruments

Q4.

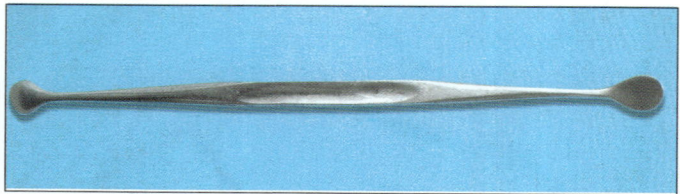

a. What is the name of the instrument?
b. What is its use?

Q5.

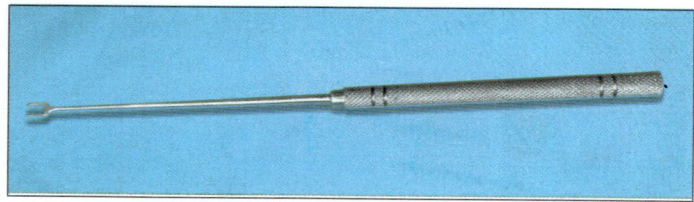

a. What is the name of the instrument?
b. What is its use?

Q6.

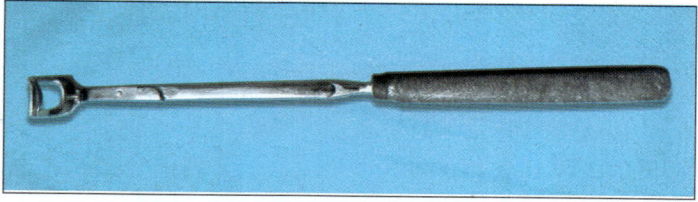

a. What is the name of the instrument?
b. What is its use?

Q7.

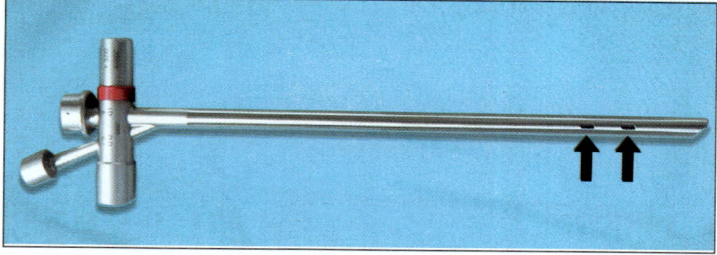

a. What is the name of the instrument?
b. What is its use?
c. What is the importance of the areas marked with arrows?

CHAPTER 19: OT Instruments

Q8.

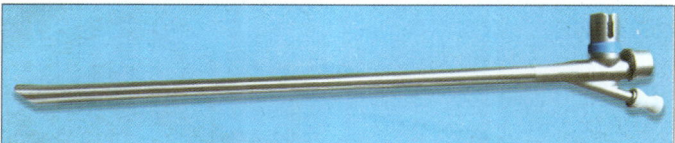

a. What is the name of the instrument?
b. What is its use?

Q9.

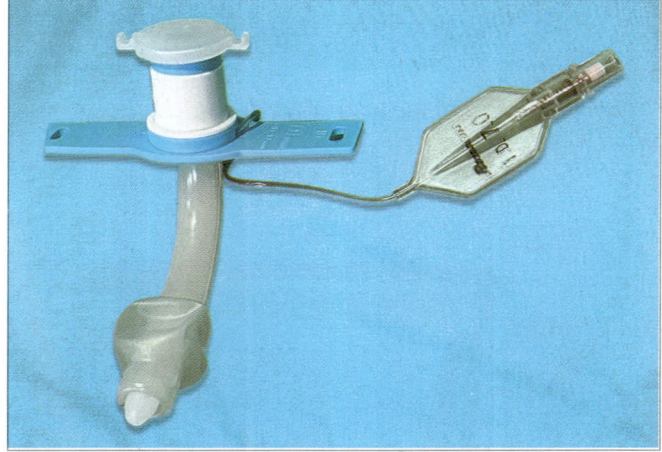

a. What is the name of the instrument?
b. What is its advantage over the metallic tubes?
c. What is the part marked with the arrow known as?

Q10.

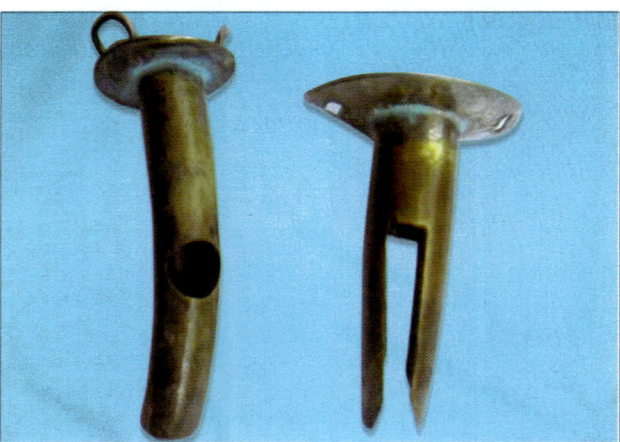

a. What is the name of the instrument?
b. What is its use?

Q11.

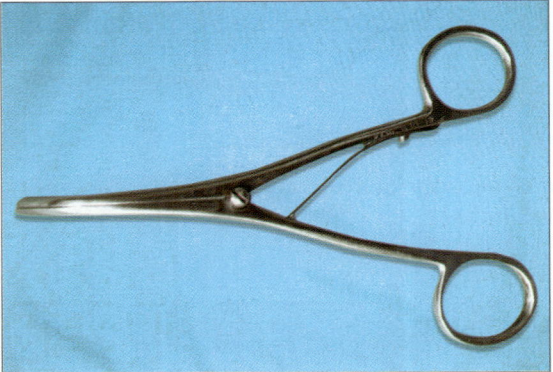

a. What is the name of the instrument?
b. What is its use?

Q12.

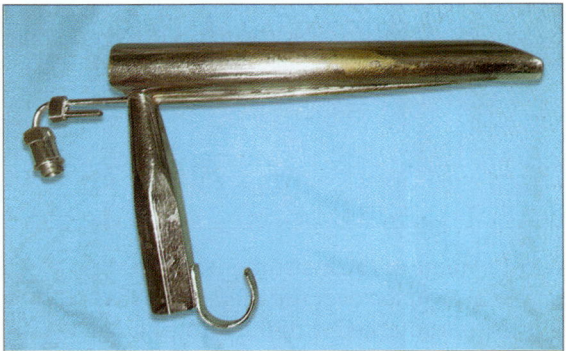

a. What is the name of the instrument?
b. What is its use?

CHAPTER 19: OT Instruments

ANSWERS

GENERAL

Ans 1:
- a. Microscope
- b. 6-40x range of magnification
- c. Ear: 200 mm, Nose: 300 mm, Throat: 400 mm

Ans 2:
- a. Endotracheal tube
- b. Used for endotracheal intubation for administering general anesthesia for surgery

Ans 3:
- a. A: 0 degree (GREEN)
  B: 30 degree (RED)
  C: 70 degree (YELLOW)
- b. 4 mm diameter

EAR SURGERY

Ans 1:
- a. Lempert's endaural speculum
- b. Used for giving canal infiltration, making canal incisions in endaural approach

Ans 2:
- a. Mollison self-retaining hemostatic mastoid retractor (3 × 3 prongs)
- b. (i) Used in tympanoplasty, mastoidectomy
  (ii) Harvesting temporalis fascia graft

Ans 3:
- a. Farabeuf mastoid periosteal elevator
- b. (i) To elevate periosteum over mastoid bone in mastoidectomy
  (ii) To elevate soft tissue and periosteum during Caldwell-Luc operation

Ans 4:
- a. A, B—Cutting burrs
  C—Diamond burr
- b. Mastoidectomy

NASAL SURGERY

Ans 1:
- a. Freer's double-ended mucoperichondrial elevator
- b. **Uses:** (i) For raising mucoperichondrial/mucoperiosteal flap in septoplasty/SMR
  (ii) For spreading and teasing the temporalis fascia graft

Ans 2:
- a. Killian long-bladed nasal speculum
- b. Anterior rhinoscopy, in nasal surgeries like septoplasty, SMR, removal of foreign bodies

Ans 3:
- a. Luc's forceps
- b. (i) Biopsy from oral cavity/oropharynx
  (ii) SMR/septoplasty for removal of cartilage or bone

Ans 4:
- a. Blakesley forceps
- b. For obtaining biopsy, during FESS/endoscopic nasal surgeries

Ans 5:
- a. Walsham forceps
- b. To correct the fractured nasal bones

Ans 6:
- a. Asch forceps
- b. Used to elevate and straighten the septum in fracture nasal septum

CHAPTER 19: OT Instruments

THROAT/OROPHARYNGEAL SURGERY

Ans 1:
  a. Boyle Davis mouth gag with tongue blade
  b. **Use:** To keep the mouth open and push the tongue up and away from the operation site in surgeries like tonsillectomy, adenoidectomy, surgeries of palate and nasopharynx

Ans 2:
  a. Dennis-Browne tonsil holding forceps
  b. To hold the tonsil and pull it medially during the process of dissection
  This instrument resembles the Luc's forcep but has some distinct differences:

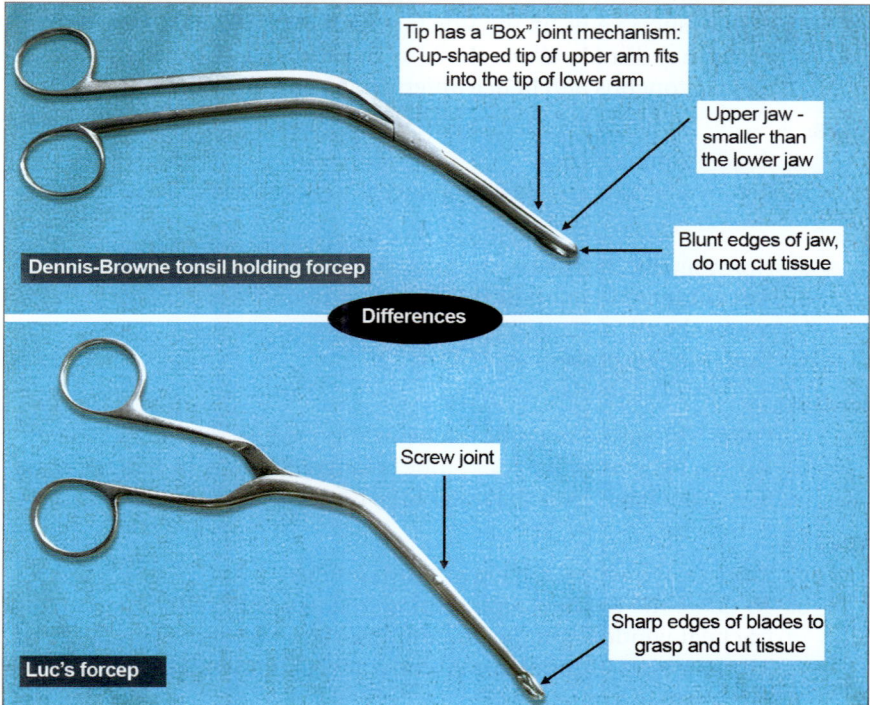

Ans 3:
  a. Negus second artery forceps
  b. Used after first artery forceps for ligating blood vessels in a deep site. The curve may be 'T' and 'J' shaped

Ans 4:
  a. Tonsillar dissector
  b. For atraumatic dissection of the tonsil from the tonsillar bed

Ans 5:
   a. Negus knot tier and ligature pusher
   b. Used to push the ligature loop on the Negus second artery forceps to ligate the bleeding point

Ans 6:
   a. St. Clair Thompson adenoid curette with cage
   b. Used to curette adenoids by a blind technique. Cage prevents slipping of the excised tissue into the throat

Ans 7:
   a. Rigid bronchoscope
   b. To perform diagnostic bronchoscopy, bronchial lavage from secretions, removal of foreign bodies from the airway
   c. Arrows show vents on the side for ventilation of the other bronchus when they remain above the level of carina when inserted into the major bronchus and hence differs from esophagoscope

Ans 8:
   a. Rigid esophagoscope
   b. Removal of foreign body, esophageal stenting, esophageal stenting

Ans 9:
   a. Non-metallic, tracheostomy tube, single-lumen, cuffed (size 7.0 mm)
   b. **Advantage:** Made up of soft material, hence less damaging to the tracheal wall
   c. **Cuff:** It helps prevent aspiration

Ans 10:
   a. Fuller's bi-valved metallic tracheostomy tube
   b. For tracheostomy, the inner tube is longer than the bi-flanged outer tube, which prevents the outer tube from getting blocked

Ans 11:
   a. Trousseau tracheal dilator with two prongs
   b. To dilate the tracheostoma during tracheostomy, after creating the tracheal window and just before inserting the tracheostomy tube. Allows easier introduction of the tracheostomy tube and prevents formation of a false passage

Ans 12:
   a. Direct laryngoscope with light carrier
   b. To take biopsy from laryngeal tumors, for excision of vocal cord polyps or cysts in Micro Laryngeal Surgery (MLS)

IMAGING

Section Outline

20. X-rays in ENT
21. Miscellaneous Imaging

X-rays in ENT

Q1. The patient was a 20-year-old male who presented with the history of trauma:

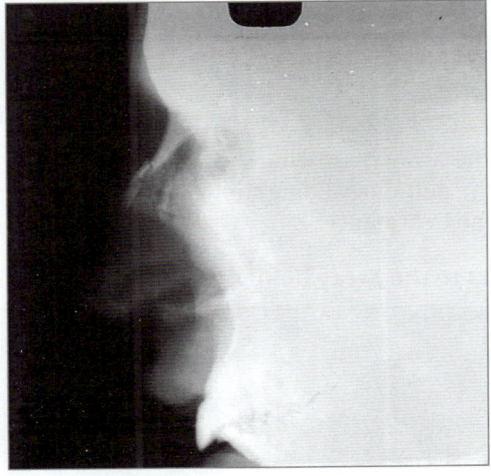

a. Identify the X-ray view.
b. What is the pathology shown here?

SECTION 6: Imaging

Q2. With respect to the X-ray below, answer the following:

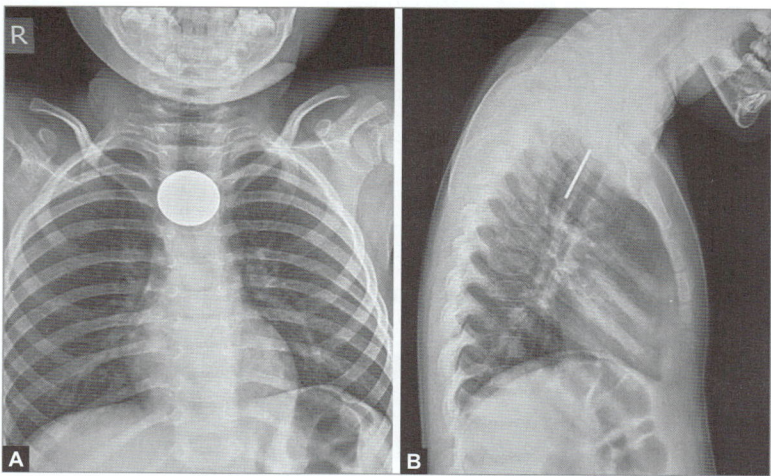

a. Identify the X-ray view being shown in Figure B.
b. What is the pathology being shown here?
c. What is the treatment?

Q3. With respect to the X-ray below, answer the following:

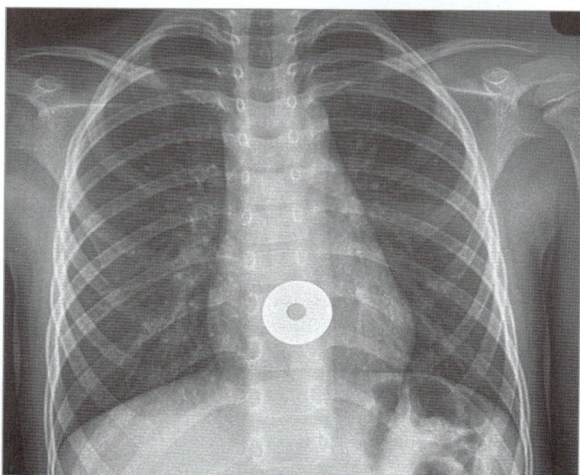

a. Identify the X-ray view being shown here.
b. What is the pathology being shown here?
c. What is the treatment?

Q4. The following is the radiograph of a child who presented with stridor and respiratory distress:

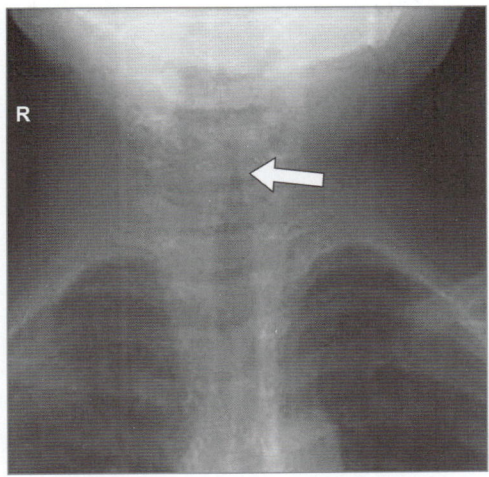

a. Name the sign being shown in the X-ray here?
b. What is the disease entity in the child that has caused this?
c. What is the causative organism of this disease?

Q5. The following is the radiograph of a toxic child who presented with inspiratory stridor, drooling and muffled voice:

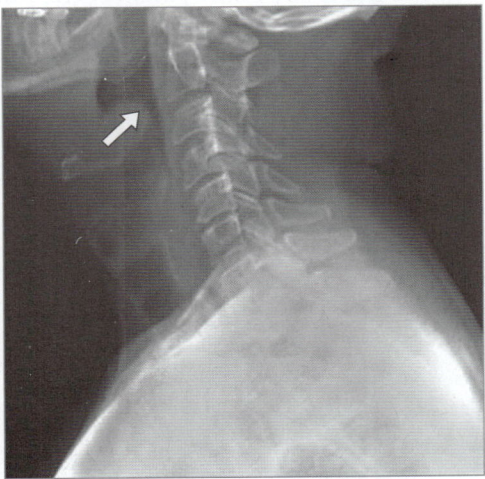

a. Name the sign being shown in the X-ray here?
b. What is the disease entity in the child that has caused this?
c. What is the causative organism of this disease?
d. What treatment will you administer?
e. What is contraindicated in a child with this suspected disease?

Q6. The following is a barium swallow of a 3-year-old boy with a history of difficulty swallowing:

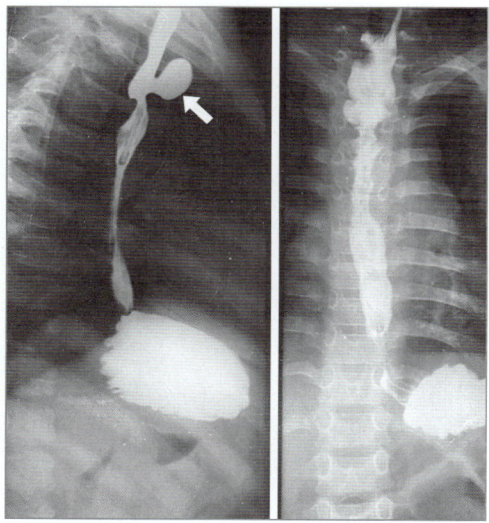

a. What is the name of the condition as pointed out by the arrow?
b. Name the defect giving rise to the above pathology.
c. What is the treatment?

Q7. With reference to the X-ray below, answer the following:

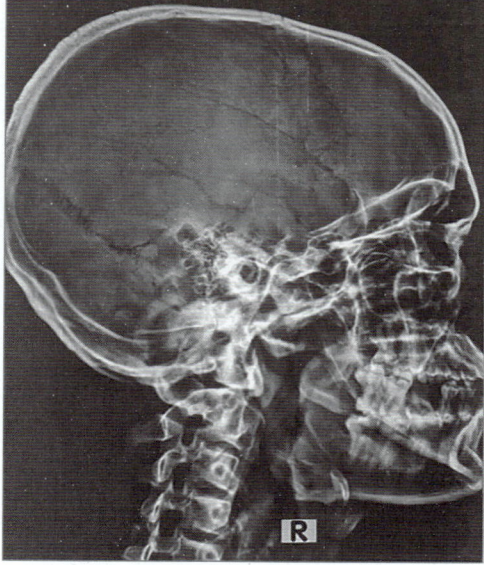

a. What is the X-ray view shown above?
b. Name three structures that this X-ray view can be used to observe.

Q8. A 5-year-old boy presented with a history of accidental ingestion of some object while playing with his brother. The following is his X-ray:

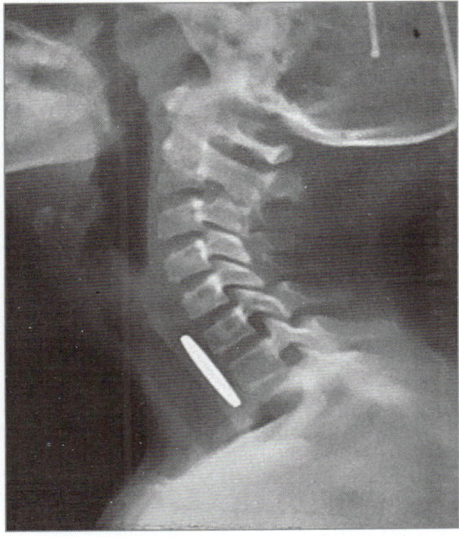

a. Identify the X-ray view being shown here.
b. What is the pathology being shown here?
c. What is the treatment?

Q9. The following is an X-ray of a patient with complaint of left sided cheek swelling:

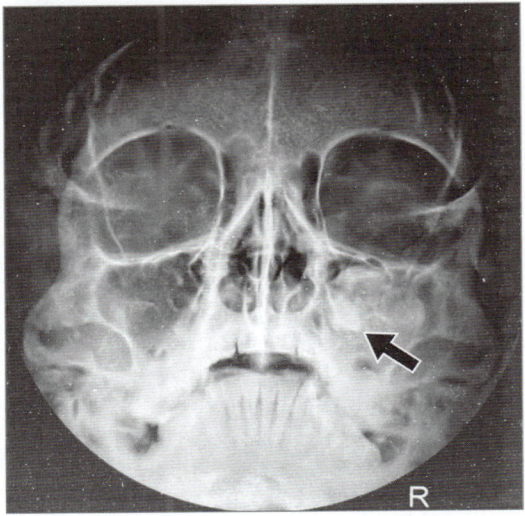

a. What is the X-ray view shown above?
b. What is its use?
c. What is the pathology shown in the X-ray?

Q10. An 8-year-old boy was brought by the father to the ENT OPD with the complaint of decreased scholastic performance. The following was his X-ray:

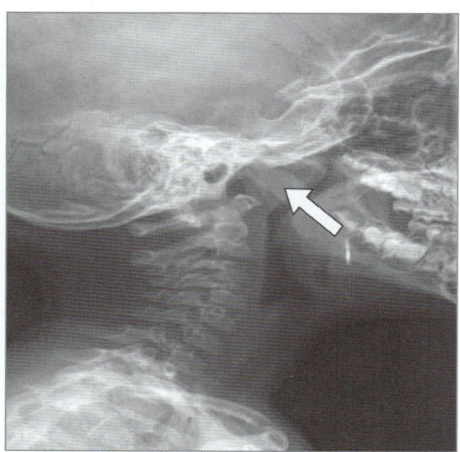

a. Why was this X-ray ordered for the child (to reach to what diagnosis)?
b. What is this X-ray view?
c. What treatment will you give the child?

Q11. The following is showing a radiograph of a patient with complaint of dysphagia:

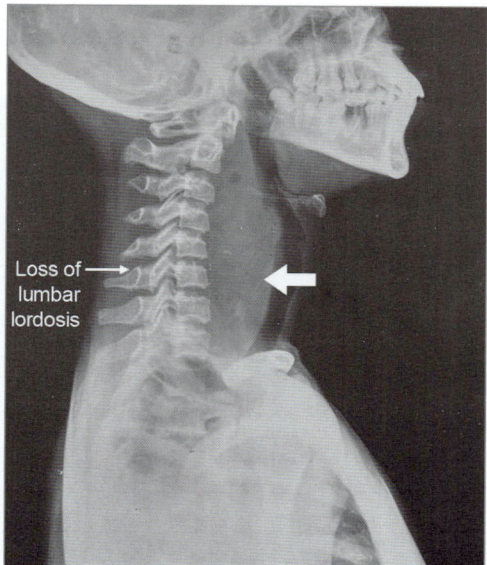

a. Identify the X-ray view shown here.
b. What is the pathology being shown here with the arrow?
c. What is the treatment?

Q12. Observe the following X-ray:

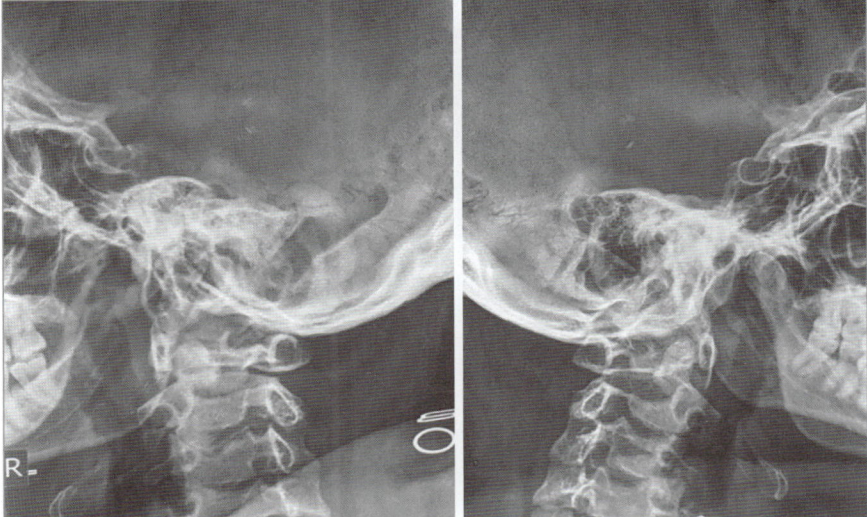

a. Identify the X-ray view shown here.
b. What is the pathology being shown?

Q13. The following is showing an X-ray AP view of a child aged 3 years:

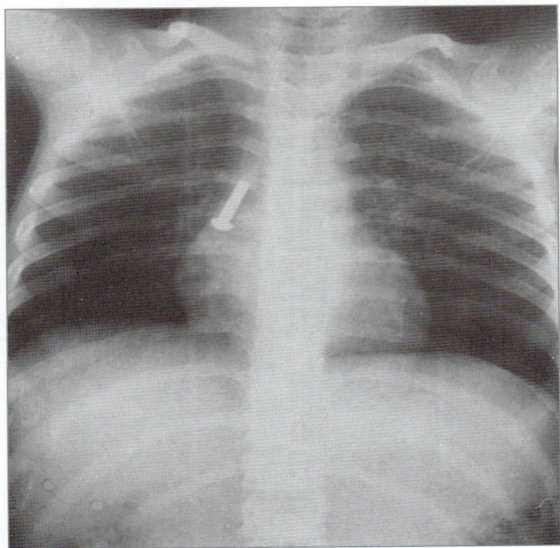

a. Identify the pathology being shown in the X-ray here.
b. What is the treatment?

Q14. The following is showing a barium swallow of a patient with a history of dysphagia (more to liquids than to solids):

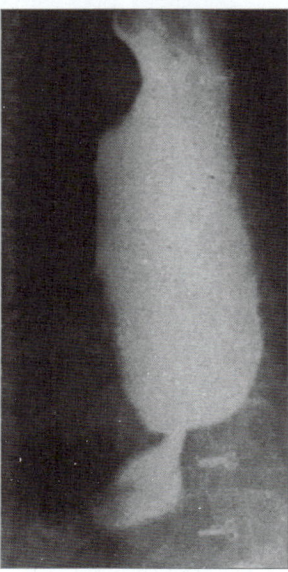

    a. Identify the pathology being shown here.
    b. What is the cause of this condition?
    c. What is the treatment of choice?

Q15. The following is showing a barium swallow of a patient with a history of dysphagia (more to solids than to liquids):

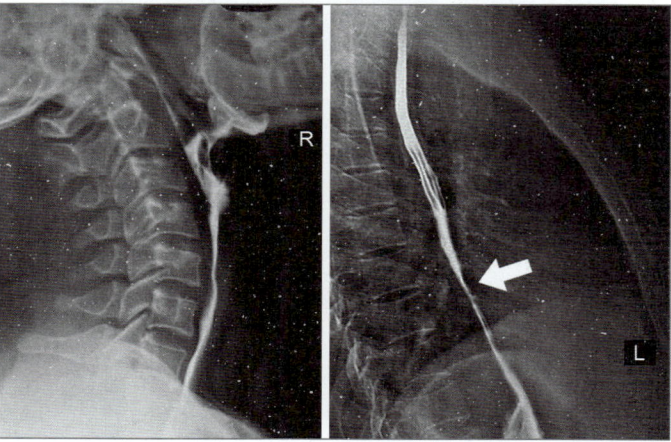

    a. Identify the pathology being shown here.
    b. Name one syndrome that can predispose to this condition?
    c. Name one investigation you should order for this patient next?

Q16. The following radiograph is of a 16-year-old lady with a persistent discharging sinus:

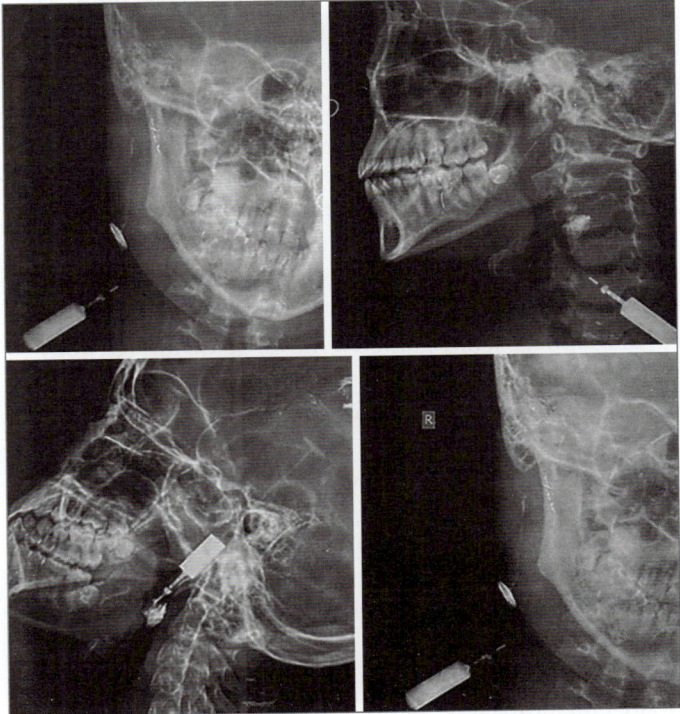

a. What is the investigation being done here?
b. Name one condition in which this is done.

ANSWERS

Ans 1:
  a. Digital X-ray nasal bone (lateral view)
  b. Fracture nasal bone

Ans 2:
  a. Digital X-ray chest (lateral view)
  b. Foreign body esophagus
  c. Rigid esophagoscopy guided removal of the foreign body

Ans 3:
  a. Digital X-ray chest (PA view)
  b. Foreign body esophagus
  c. Rigid esophagoscopy guided removal of the foreign body

Ans 4:
  a. 'Steeple' sign/'Pencil-tip' sign: Narrowing of the subglottic airway owing to mucosal edema in croup (Subglottis being the narrowest portion of the pediatric airway, its edema causes the critical symptom of stridor)
  b. Acute laryngotracheobronchitis/croup
  c. Parainfluenza virus (type 1: mainly, type 2, type 3: sometimes), respiratory syncytial virus (RSV) type A and B, Rhinovirus

Ans 5:
  a. 'Thumb' sign
  b. Acute epiglottitis
  c. Invasive *Haemophilus influenzae b* (traditionally). In postvaccination era, may be due to 'vaccination breakthrough', *meningococci*, group A *streptococci, pneumococci*, etc.
  d. Intravenous antibiotics (empirical with third generation cephalosporins for 5–7 days, due to ampicillin resistance in over 50% in *Haemophilus influenzae*)
  e. When acute epiglottitis is suspected, pharyngeal examination should not be attempted, as simple manipulation with a tongue depressor may precipitate acute obstruction. If it is to be done, controlled setting should be available (like pediatric intensive care unit)

Ans 6:
  a. Zenker's diverticulum
  b. Killian's dehiscence—a weak area between the two parts of the inferior constrictor muscle
  c. Treatment:
      i. Excision of the pouch and cricopharyngeal myotomy
      ii. Dohlman's procedure
      iii. Endoscopic laser treatment

Ans 7:
a. Digital X-ray mastoid (lateral oblique view or Law's view)
b. Structures seen:
   i. Mastoid air calls (extent of pneumatization)
   ii. Tegmen
   iii. Sinus plate

Ans 8:
a. Digital X-ray soft tissue lateral neck
b. Foreign body esophagus
c. Rigid esophagoscopy guided removal of the foreign body

Ans 9:
a. Digital X-ray of paranasal sinuses (Water's view)
b. To see the structures like: Maxillary sinus (best seen), frontal sinuses, sphenoid sinus (if film is taken with mouth open), zygoma, zygomatic arch, nasal bone, frontal process of maxilla, superior orbital fissure, infratemporal fossa
c. Left maxillary dentigerous cyst

Ans 10:
a. To check for adenoid hypertrophy
b. Digital X-ray soft tissue lateral neck (neck extended)
c. Initially conservative, topical steroid nasal sprays, anti-histaminics, decongestant nasal drops

Ans 11:
a. Digital X-ray soft tissue lateral neck
b. Retropharyngeal abscess, showing widening of the prevertebral space
c. **Treatment:** Initially, high-dose intravenous antibiotics. If pus collection is suspected, urgent incision and drainage is done under a general anesthetic by an experienced anesthetist. Drainage is usually done per-orally, but occasionally external drainage via neck may be appropriate. Very rarely, tracheostomy might be required. Retropharyngeal abscess due to tuberculosis requires specific antibiotic treatment

Ans 12:
a. Digital X-ray mastoid (lateral oblique view or Law's view/Schuller's view)
b. Mastoiditis (right)

Ans 13:
a. Foreign body right bronchus
b. Rigid bronchoscopy guided removal of foreign body

Ans 14:
   a. Megaesophagus (achalasia cardia)
   b. Failure of the lower esophageal sphincter to relax with dilatation of esophagus due to stasis of food due to degeneration of ganglion cells of Auerbach's plexus
   c. Modified Heller's operation (myotomy of the narrowed lower portion of the esophagus)

Ans 15:
   a. Irregular filling defect in the lower part of the esophagus – probably due to carcinoma esophagus
   b. Plummer-Vinson syndrome
   c. CECT neck, thorax, abdomen – to assess the extent of the disease, nodal metastases, status of vessels, etc.

Ans 16:
   a. Fistulogram
   b. Branchial fistula

Miscellaneous Imaging

Q1. The following is a high-resolution computed tomography (HRCT) of the temporal bone. Answer the following:

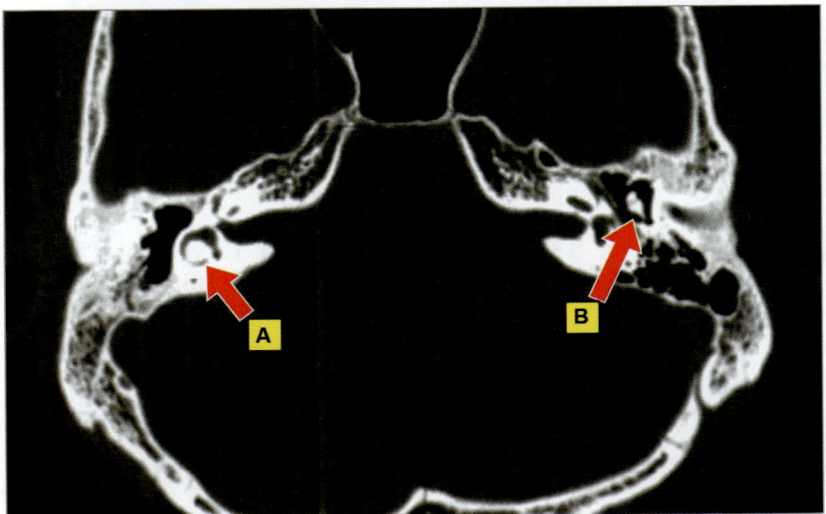

  a. Identify the 'signet-ring' like structure being shown by the arrow labelled as 'A' in the CT.
  b. The structure labelled by the arrow marked as 'B' in the figure shows the ossicles.
     Which ossicles complex is shown here, and what is the appearance called as?
  c. What is meant by "high-resolution" CT scan?

Q2. The following shows a CT scan of paranasal sinuses of a 33-year-old gentleman, with complaints of unilateral, foul-smelling nasal discharge and nasal obstruction, with "double-density" sign on the CT:

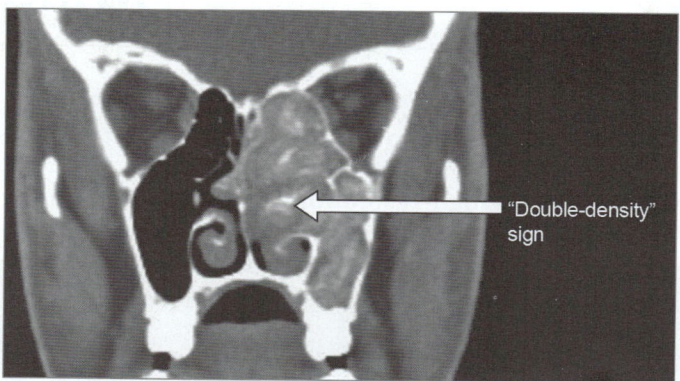

a. What is the probable diagnosis evident from the CT scan?
b. Why does "double density" sign occur?

Q3. The following is showing the MRI of a 12-year-old boy with complaint of recurrent episodes of profuse epistaxis since last one year.

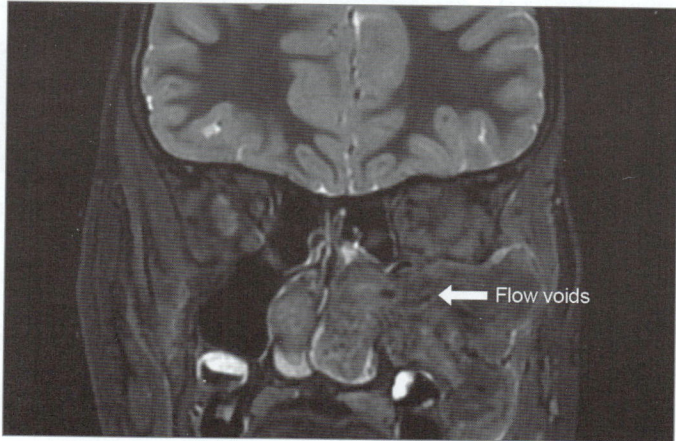

a. What is the most probable diagnosis evident from the MRI scan?
b. Mention the appearance of CSF on T1 versus T2 MRI sequences.
c. Mention one advantage of MRI over CT scan.

Q4. The following images show an imaging done in a patient with squamous cell carcinoma of the oral cavity and the larynx:

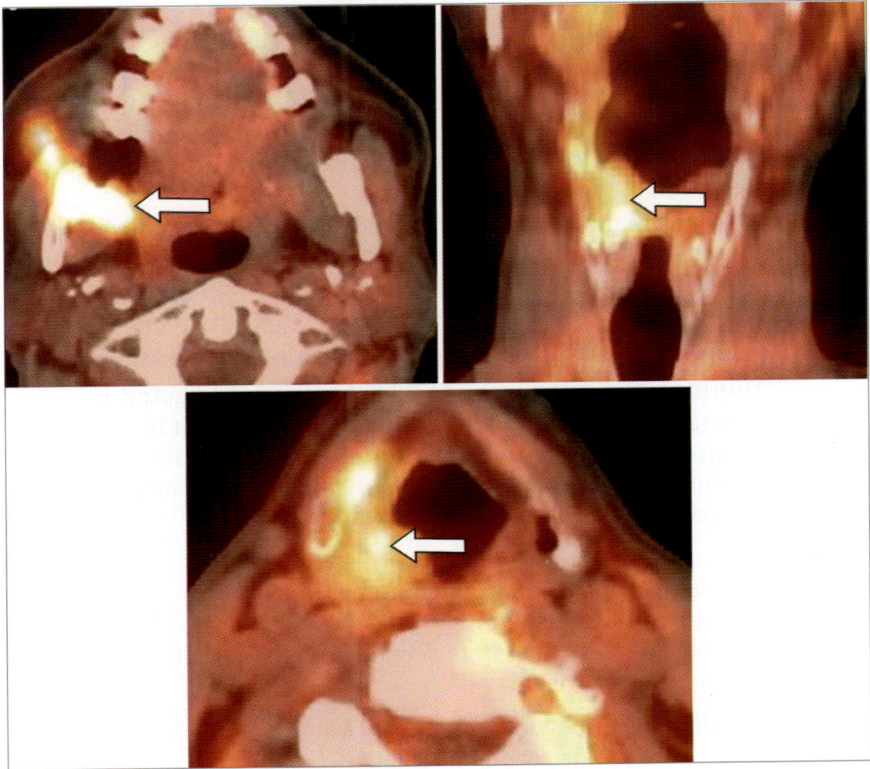

a. What is the imaging modality that is shown here?
b. Name one radiotracer substance used in this scan.
c. What is one disadvantage of this scan?

ANSWERS

Ans 1:
    a. Lateral semi-circular canal (Right side)
    b. **Incus-malleus complex** (Head of malleus and body and short process of the incus is seen). This is the level at which the representative **"cone and ice cream" appearance** of the incus-malleus complex is seen just lateral to the tympanic segment of the facial nerve
    c. CT scan with thin slices of **less than 1 mm** is called high-resolution CT scan. It allows precise demonstration of fine middle ear structures such as the ossicular chain and inner ear

Ans 2:
    a. Allergic fungal rhinosinusitis (AFRS)
    b. "Double density" sign in AFRS: Seen in the affected sinuses, heterogeneous signal intensity due to deposition of heavy metals within the allergic mucin. Hyper-attenuation of the intra-sinus contents (representing thick allergic mucin), surrounded by lower attenuation hyperplastic mucosa

Ans 3:
    a. Juvenile nasopharyngeal angiofibroma (JNA)
    b. CSF: Dark on T1; bright on T2
    c. Does not use radiation (More accurate soft tissue delineation)

Ans 4:
    a. PET (Positron emission tomography) scan
    b. 2-(F18) fluoro-2-deoxyglucose (FDG)
    c. High uptake may be seen physiologically in Brown adipose tissue or areas with inflammation and infection may also have high uptake giving false positive findings

SECTION 7

RECENT ADVANCES

Section Outline

22. Recent Advances

Recent Advances

Q1. The following is showing the zones of destruction caused by a LASER BEAM.

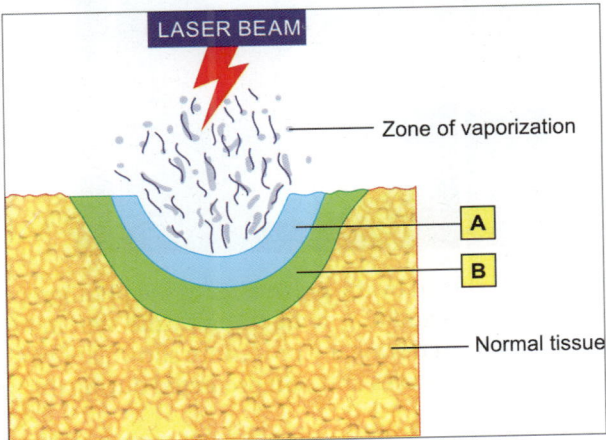

a. Label zones marked "A" and "B".
b. What is the wavelength of CO_2 laser?
c. What is the delivery system used for CO_2 LASER, as it cannot pass through optical fibers?
d. Name two LASER having wavelengths in the visible spectrum which are used in ear surgery.

Q2. The following image is showing Micro Laryngeal Surgery (MLS) being performed in the OT.

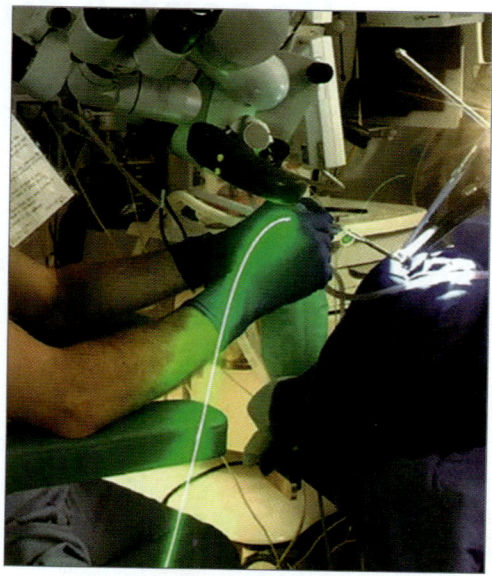

a. What is being shown by the green fiber in the photograph?
b. What specific precaution is to be taken by the staff in the operating room for their eyes during the procedure shown above?
c. How is the patient's eyes and skin protected during the procedure?

Q3. The following illustration is showing a therapy being administered to a cancer patient:

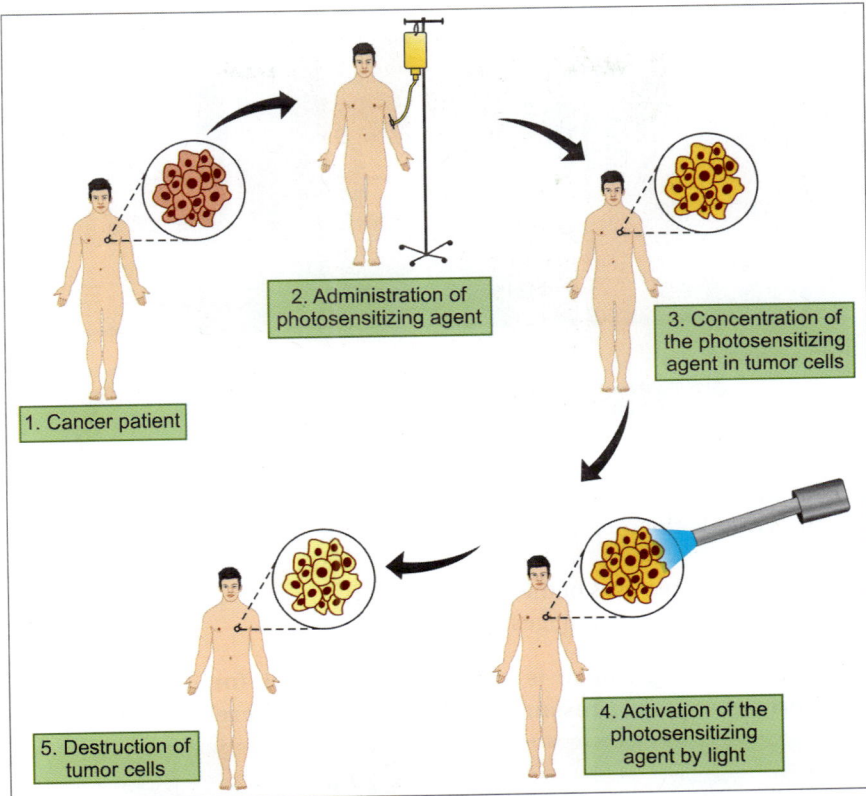

a. Identify the therapy being given in the illustration above.
b. What is the laser light used generally in this therapy?
c. Name three photosensitizing agents used for the therapy shown above.
d. What precautions should the patient take after the therapy strictly?

Q4. The following image is showing a device which generates very high-frequency electromagnetic waves to cause tissue ablation:

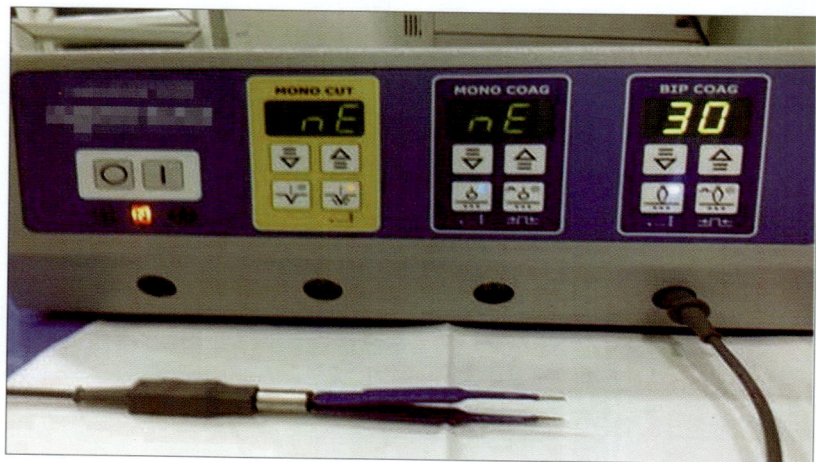

a. What is this device being shown?
b. What is the mechanism by which tissue damage is caused by this device?
c. Name three uses of this in ENT surgery.
d. What are its advantages?

Q5. The following image is showing a chamber for delivering 100 percent oxygen, pressurized above 1 atmosphere absolute (ATA):

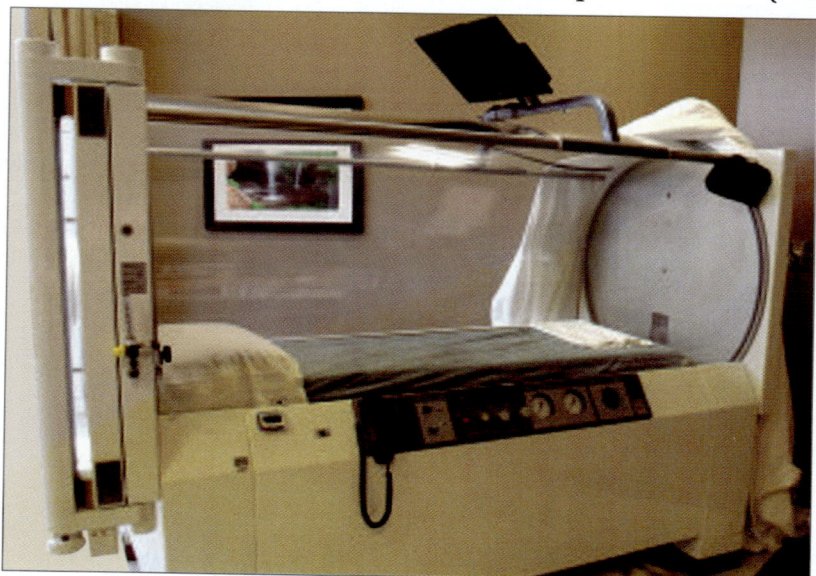

a. Identify the therapy which uses this.
b. Name two indications for which it is used in ENT.
c. What is the treatment protocol generally used?

Q6. Answer the following questions with respect to the images shown below:

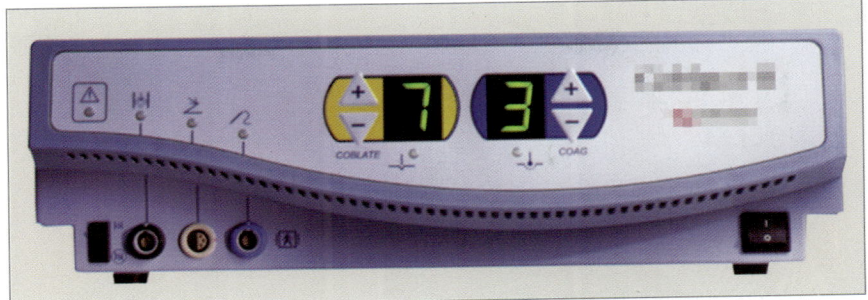

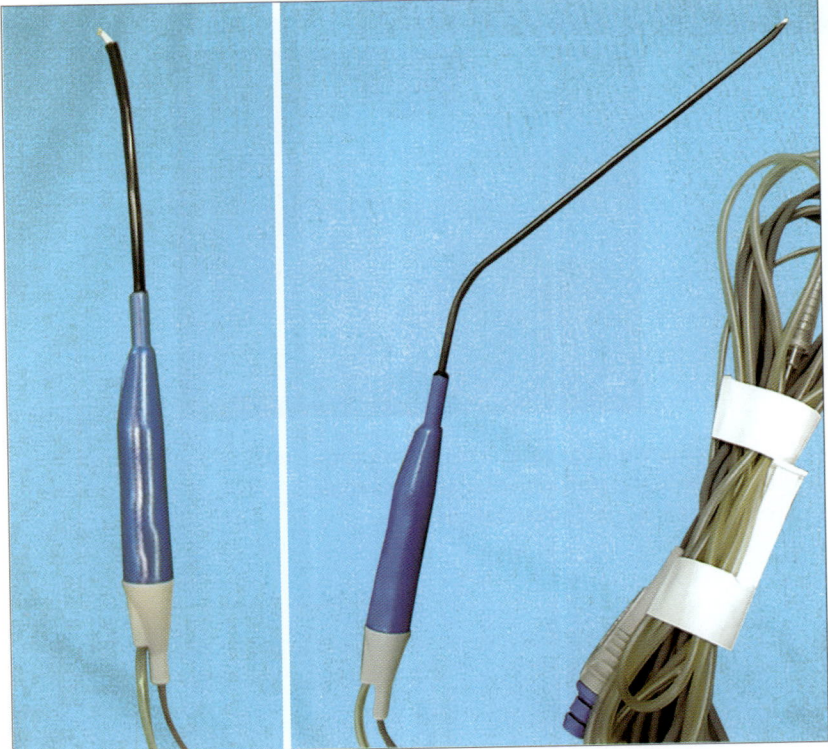

a. What is the name of the device being shown here?
b. What is the principle of the device?
c. Mention 5 uses of the device.

Q7. The following images shows a thermoplastic mask, custom-made for a patient with head and neck carcinoma:

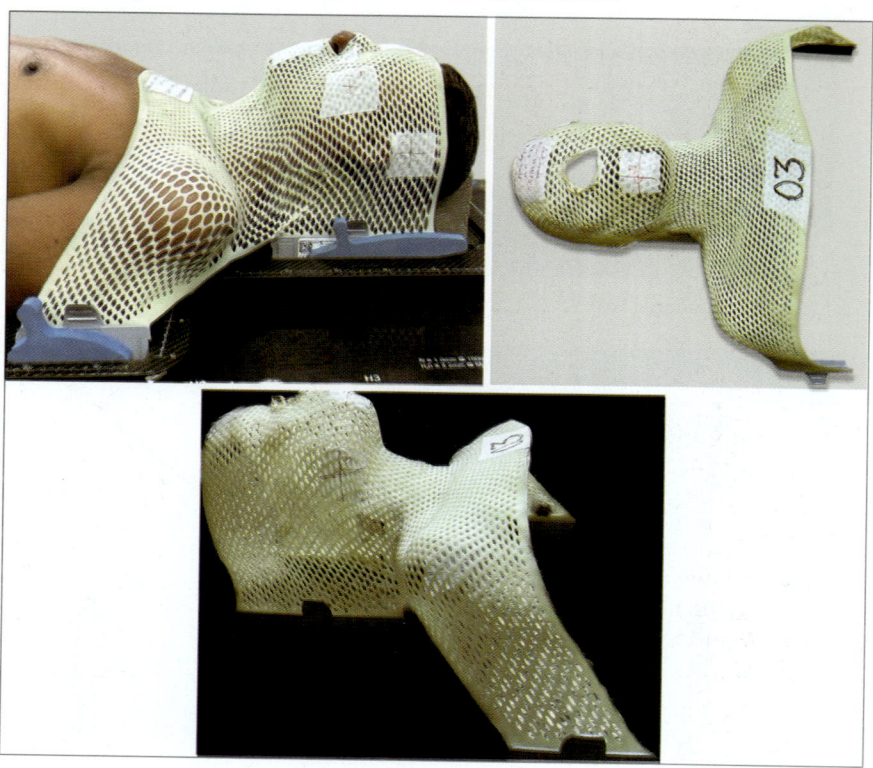

a. During what therapy is this mask required?
b. What is the purpose of using this mask?
c. What is hyperfractionation?

Q8. **Answer with respect to the images below:**

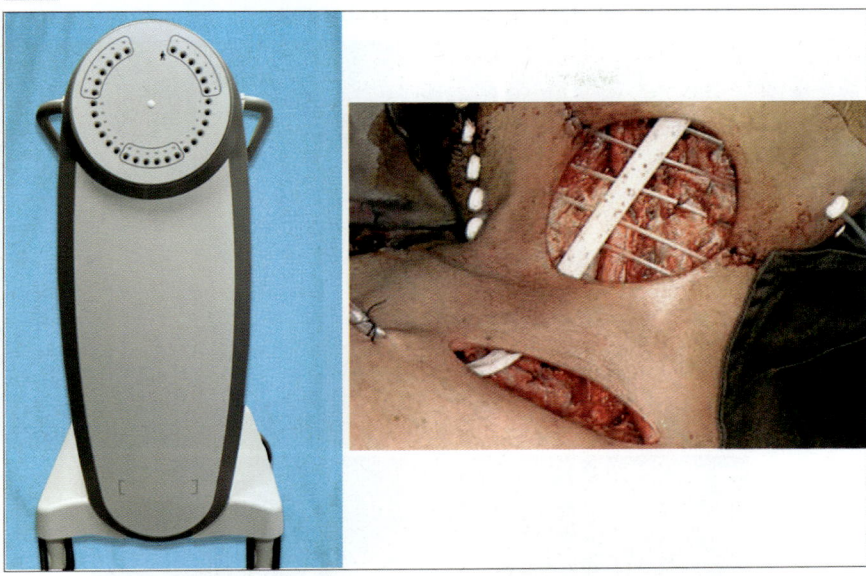

a. What is being shown in the picture above?
b. Name four materials used for the therapy being shown above.
c. Mention one advantage and one disadvantage of this.
d. Mention one dreaded complication.

Q9. The following is showing the planning imaging for the radiotherapy for a patient with carcinoma:

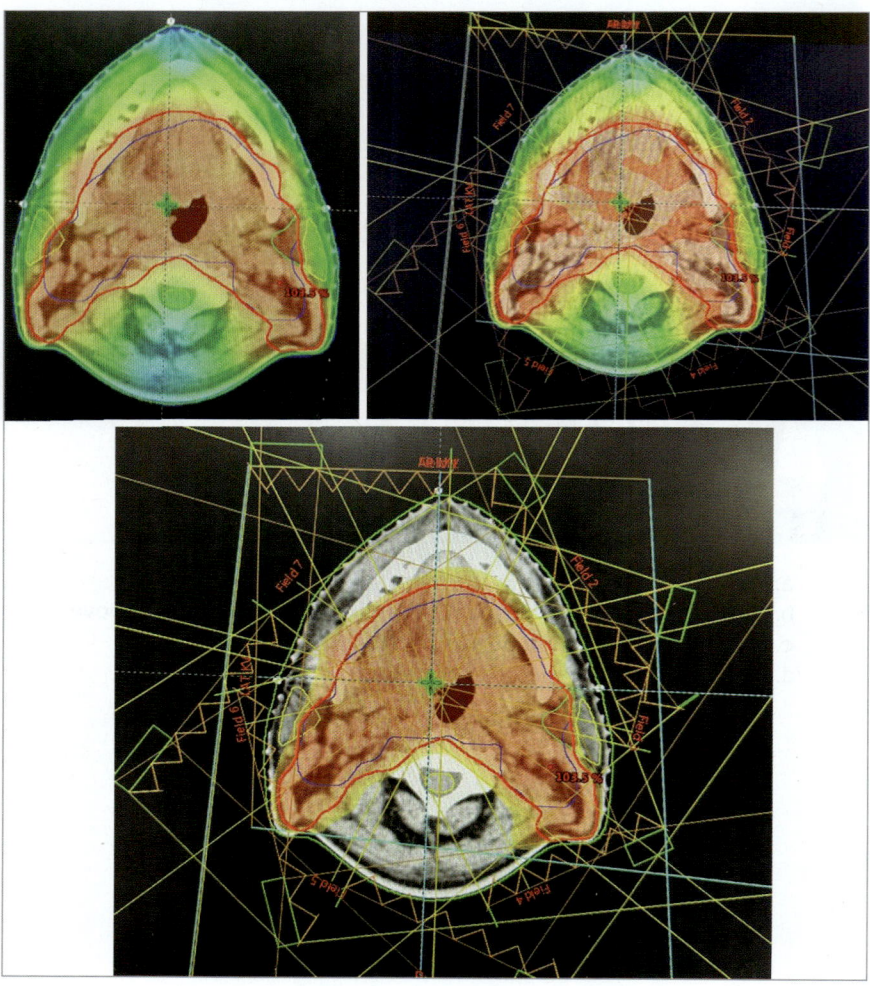

    a. What is the type of radiotherapy being planned here to be given to the patient?
    b. What is the distinct advantage of this procedure?
    c. What is the machine through which it is delivered?

Q10. The following is showing sections of the radiotherapy planning CT for a patient with carcinoma:

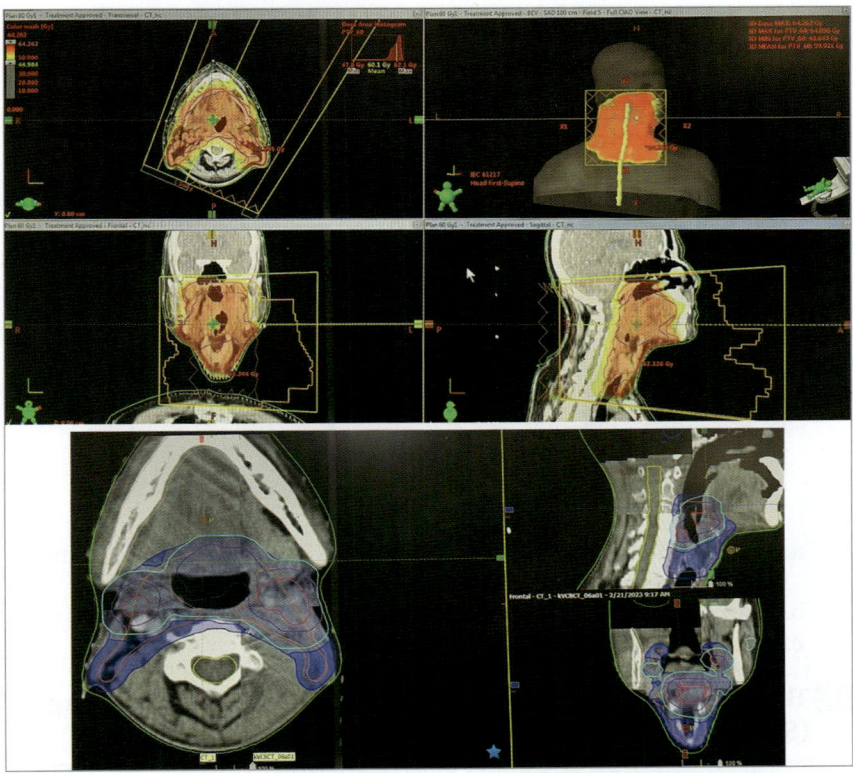

a. What does IGRT stand for?
b. What is its advantage over IMRT?
c. Mention two side effects of IMRT.

Q11. The following image shows the radiotherapy setup for delivery to patient with head/neck malignancy:

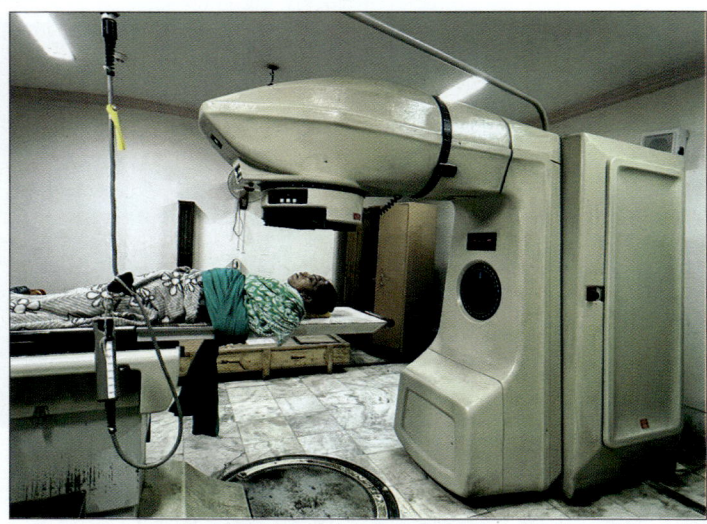

a. What is the radiotherapy modality that will be delivered in the image being shown here?
b. Name the radioactive source being used in this setup.
c. Give one disadvantage of this therapy.

Q12. The following images are related to stereotactic radiosurgery (SRS):

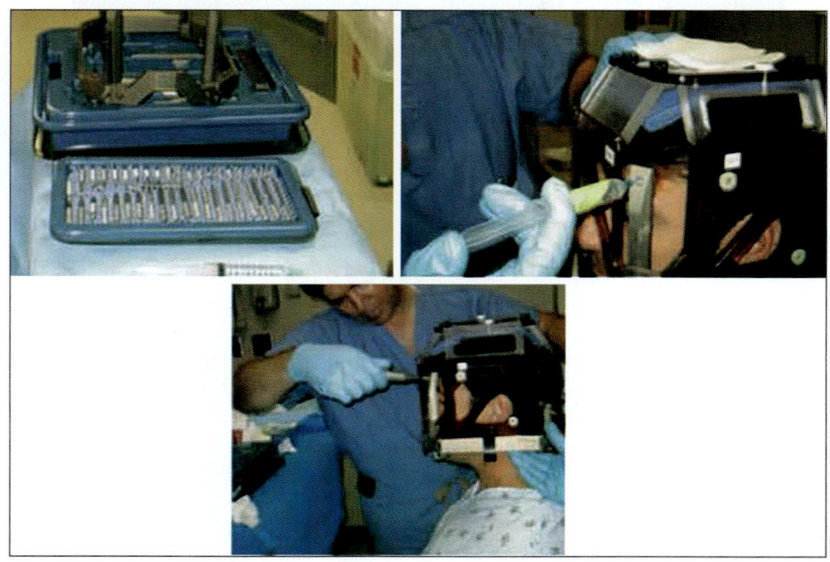

a. What is being shown in the pictures?
b. Mention one application of this type of radiotherapy.
c. What is the radiation dose generally used?

Q13. The following shows a model of a radiotherapy delivery device:

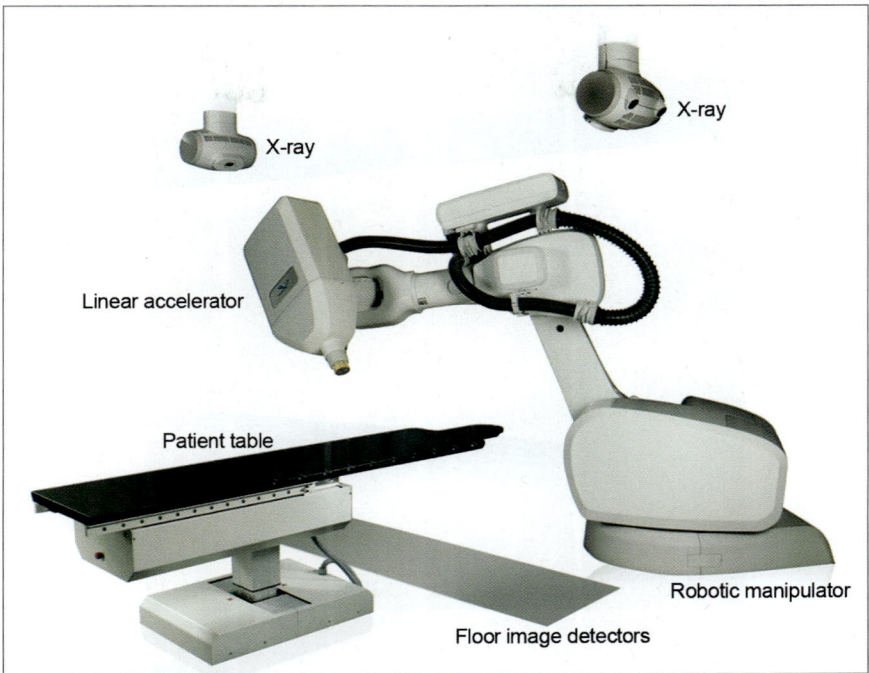

a. Name the device being shown here.
b. What are its differences with the Gamma Knife.

Q14. The following is showing surgery being performed on a patient with laryngopharyngeal cancer:

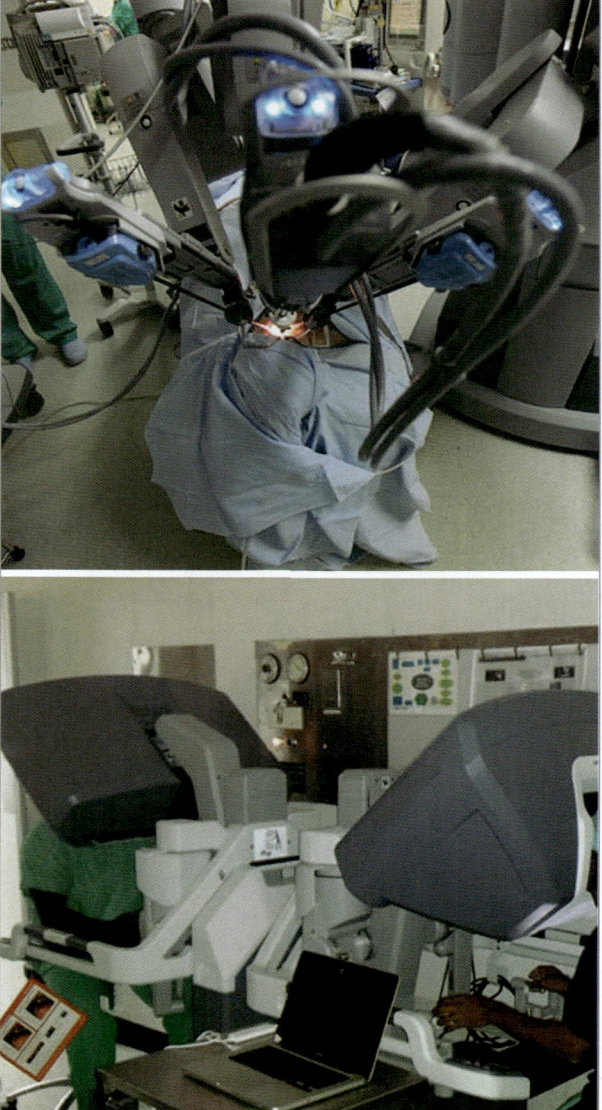

a. What is the device in use being shown here?
b. What is the advantage of this type of surgery?
c. Give one disadvantage of this type of surgery.

Q15. The following is showing the MRI of a 14-year-old boy with juvenile nasopharyngeal angiofibroma (JNA):

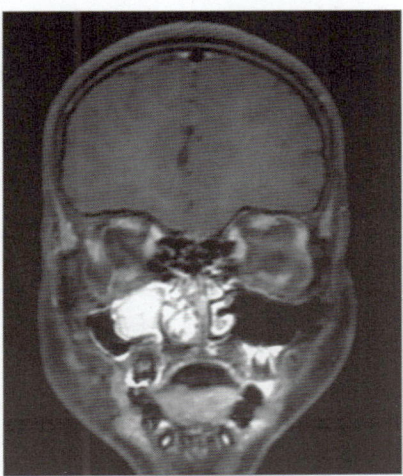

Before taking up this patient for surgery a procedure was performed by the interventional radiologist in the DSA (digital subtraction angiography) suite. The following are the pre- and post-procedure photos:

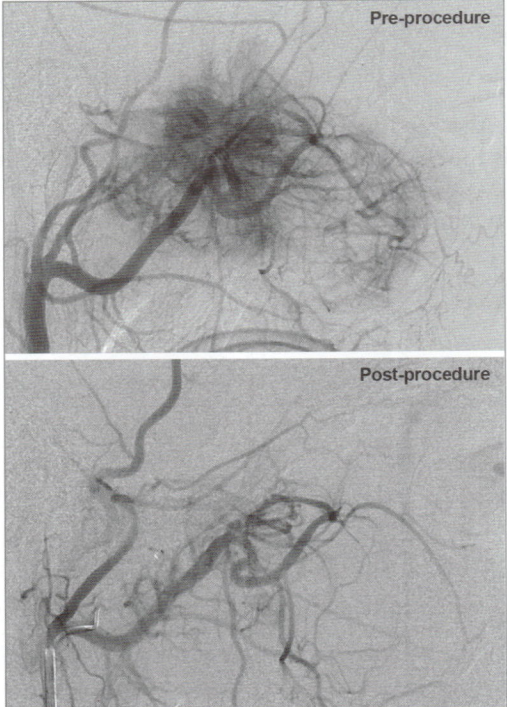

a. What is the procedure that was performed on the boy?
b. What materials can be used for the procedure?
c. Name one complication of this procedure.

Q16. The following image shows a patient with nasopharyngeal carcinoma, about to undergo IMRT treatment:

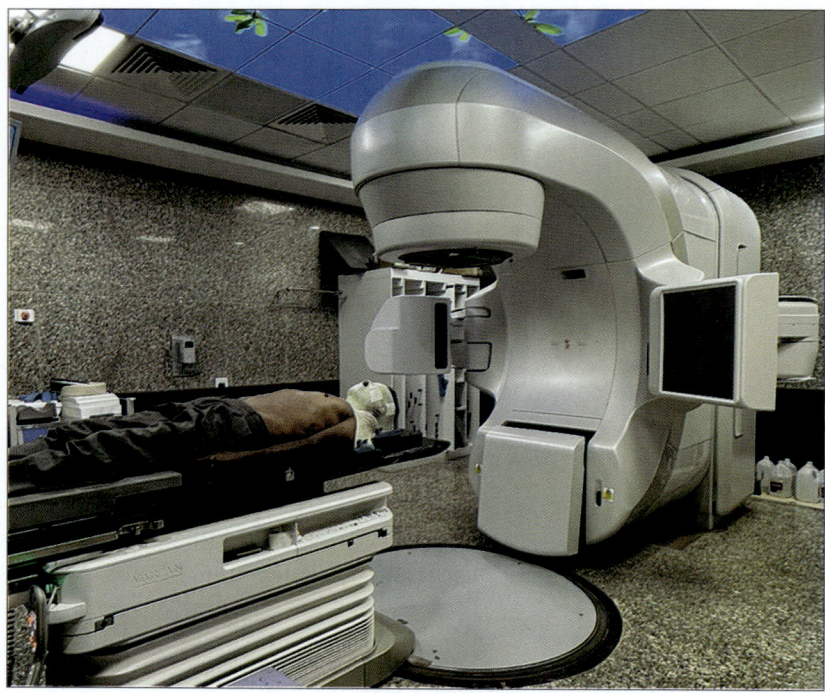

a. What is the machine shown here for delivery of the radiotherapy?
b. What is the difference between stereotactic radiotherapy (SRT) and stereotactic radiosurgery (SRS)?
c. Name two radiosensitizer agents.

Q17. The following image shows a CT scan machine that can capture the location and movement of a tumor and the movement of the body's organs over time.

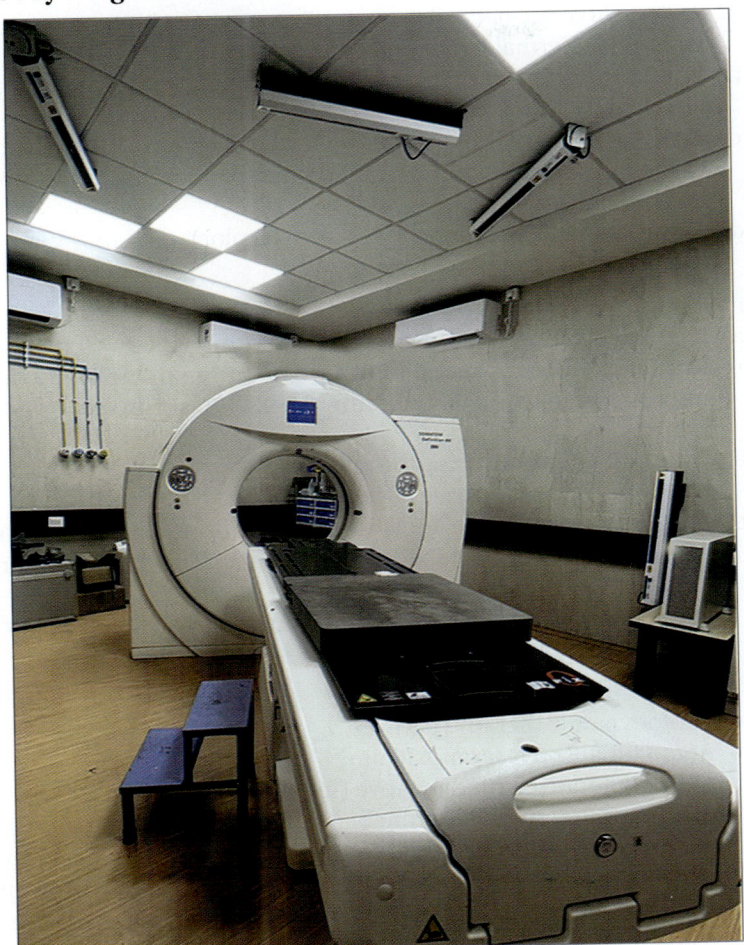

a. What is this advanced CT known as?
b. Name an endocrine disorder in which it has wide application.
c. Name one disadvantage of this CT over conventional CT.

ANSWERS

Ans 1:
a. A: Zone of tissue necrosis
   B: Zone of thermal repair and conductivity
b. 10,600 nm (invisible, hence requires an aiming bean of helium-neon laser)
c. Articulated arm with a series of reflective mirrors to direct the beam to the target area. Requires a micromanipulator if working through an operating microscope
d. Argon laser (488-514 nm, blue-green in color)
   KTP laser (532 nm)

Ans 2:
a. KTP laser being used during microlaryngoscopy. A protective shuttering filter is attached to the operating microscope during microlaryngoscopy when using the KTP laser in the operating room
b. Other personnel not using the microscope would be required to wear wave-specific protective eyewear
c. Double layer of saline-moistened eye pads are secured with silk tape. The eyes are first taped closed with silk tape to prevent corneal abrasions from the eye pads
   Saline-moistened towels are placed around the patient's head to cover all skin surfaces

Ans 3:
a. Photodynamic therapy (PDT)
b. Argon tunable dye laser (630 nm)
c. i. Hematoporphyrin derivative (for head and neck cancers)
   ii. Photosan-3 (for endobronchial tumors)
   iii. Delta-aminolevulinic acid (topical sensitizer, for skin cancers)
d. Patients receiving photodynamic therapy should avoid exposure to sunlight and use sun-protective clothing to avoid photosensitive skin reactions which may continue for several weeks

Ans 4:
   a. Radiofrequency ablation device (Radiosurg 2200, ENT Version, 2.2 MHz, Meyer Haake, Germany,) with the small conventional reusable bipolar cautery forceps
   b. Radiofrequency waves (350 kHz to 4 MHz) delivered to tissue via probe
      ➢ Ionic agitation in tissues and tissue heating (temperature between 80 to 85 degree celsius)
      ➢ Protein coagulation
      ➢ Tissue necrosis
   c. i. Reduction of inferior turbinate hypertrophy to relieve nasal obstruction
      ii. Radiofrequency ablation of tongue base in sleep apnea surgery
      iii. Correction of rhinophyma or cosmetic removal of skin lesions
   d. Minimal lateral tissue damage and charring, minimally invasive technique, can be performed as OPD procedure, cost effective

Ans 5:
   a. Hyperbaric oxygen therapy (HBOT)
   b. i. Sudden sensorineural hearing loss (SSNHL)—Patients with moderate to profound SSNHL (more than or equal to 41dB) presenting within 14 days of onset of symptoms
      ii. Malignant otitis externa (to bring about healing)
   c. 100% oxygen at (2.0 – 2.5) ATA for 90 minutes daily for 10–20 treatments

Ans 6:
   a. Coblator II surgery system using patented coblation technology
   b. Radiofrequency energy passed through saline
      ➢ Ionization of high-energy sodium ad chloride ions in the saline
      ➢ Creation of plasma field of energy
      ➢ Breaks organic molecular bonds of soft tissues
      ➢ Tissue dissolution at low temperature (40–70°C)

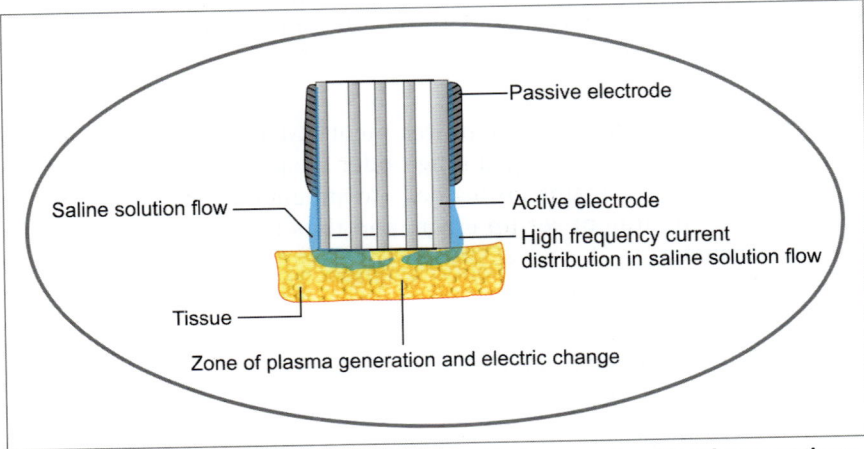

Mechanism of tissue damage at the area of the coblation wand touching the target tissue

c. 5 uses:
   i. Adenotonsillectomy
   ii. Laryngeal papillomas
   iii. Tongue base reduction
   iv. Kashima operation (transverse cordectomy) for bilateral abductor paralysis
   v. Juvenile nasopharyngeal angiofibroma (JNA) excision

Ans 7:
   a. Radiotherapy for head-neck cancer treatment (Three-dimensional conformal radiotherapy or 3D-CRT, IMT, IGRT, etc.)
   b. It is an immobilization shell, used so that the patient's position remains stable during delivery of the radiation
   c. Hyperfractionation: Delivering multiple daily doses of radiotherapy in such a way that the overall treatment time remains the same as in conventional radiotherapy. Dose of each fraction is typically reduced to 1.1–1.2 Gy/fraction, and 2 fractions/day are given. So, a higher total dose of nearly 74–870 Gy can be delivered in about the same treatment duration

Ans 8:
   a. Brachytherapy ["Brachy" *(Greek)* – Means 'short'; form of radiotherapy where a sealed radiation source is placed inside or close to the tumor, delivery of the radiotherapy done via thin tubes called catheters]
   b. Iridium (^{192}Ir), Radium (^{226}Ra), Cesium (^{137}Cs), Gold (^{198}Au)
   c. One advantage—better dose localization, less radiation damage to surrounding healthy tissue, rapid dose fall-off away from the source
   One disadvantage—generally invasive, may require general anesthesia (also does not address subclinical disease)
   d. Osteoradionecrosis

Ans 9:
   a. Intensity modulated radiotherapy treatment (IMRT)
   b. Minimizes radiation to surrounding normal structures
   c. Linear accelerator

Ans 10:
   a. Image guided radiotherapy treatment (IGRT)
   b. It is basically IMRT planning under image guidance done on the treatment machine during daily treatment delivery. It reduces the daily treatment set-up errors and thus has more precision and accuracy
   c. Xerostomia, mucositis

Ans 11:
   a. EBRT (External Beam Radio Therapy)
   b. Cobalt sources (Co60)
   c. Xerostomia

Ans 12:

a. Stereotactic head frame with MRI fiducial box placement before SRS
   The MRI fiducial box is used with the stereotactic head frame to provide fiducial markers (or reference points) in the image to position the patient's brain in the stereotactic coordinate system. The MR images are then sent to the treatment planning software to obtain the stereotactic target coordinates x, y and z before the SRS
b. Acoustic neuroma
c. For small acoustic neuromas (<3 cm)—treated by SRS alone (dose of 12–14 Gy in a single session); for largers tumors- generally surgery first followed by radiation with conventional dose of 50 Gy in 5 weeks

Ans 13:

a. Cyberknife
b. Differences:

Cyberknife	Gamma knife
Non-invasive (Patient wears a soft, mesh mask during treatment)	Invasive (Patient wears a large, metal head frame that is bolted into the skull)
Accuracy enabled by advanced robotics intelligent tumor tracking and real-time imaging	Accuracy enabled by keeping patient immobilized during treatment
Flexible treatment options, single high dose treatment or two to five low dose treatments, generally completed within a week	Due to invasive head frame, patients are limited to single high dose treatment, from fixed angles
Use of electrically generated photons to treat	Use of radioactive cobalt to treat
Anesthesia not required	Local anesthesia required for fixing pins of head frame
Treats tumors throughout body (stereotactic radiosurgery – SRS or stereotactic body radiation therapy – SBRT or stereotactic ablative radiotherapy –SABR)	Limited to tumor treatment in the skull and selected cases in cervical spine
Radiation delivery through thousands of angles	Radiation delivery through a limited number of angles

Cyberknife

Gamma knife

Ans 14:
- a. Robotic surgery (The da Vinci surgical system (Intuitive Surgical Inc., Sunnyvale, CA) is being shown here. The robotic system is seen to be docked in the mouth for performing the transoral robotic surgery (TORS) for laryngopharyngeal cancer)
- b. Increased surgical precision by eliminating tremors and fatigue by motion scaling, telesurgery possible, telemonitoring possible, better vision possible
- c. High cost, lack of tactile feedback

Ans 15:
- a. Pre-operative embolization of JNA to reduce vascularity of tumor and reduce intra-operative bleeding)
- b. Polyvinyl alcohol particles (PVA), Trisacryl gelatin particles, coils, balloons, Cyanoacrylate adhesives (NBCA), Ethylene vinyl alcohol copolymer (Onyx)
- c. Blindness (Due to emboli to ophthalmic artery), Hemiplegia, etc.

Ans 16:
- a. LINAC (linear accelerator – can produce high-energy X-rays, in the range of Megaelectron-volts (MeV))
- b. **SRT:** Radiotherapy given in fractions
  SRS: Radiotherapy given in single session (uses head frame, which is invasively fixed using anesthesia), e.g., Used in acoustic neuroma (<3 cm)
- c. Radiosensitizers—agents which assist in making the radiation become more effective; sensitizing cells to the radiotherapy. They act by: (1) reducing hypoxia, (2) giving concomitant chemotherapy, and (3) giving targeted therapy
  Examples: Hyperbaric oxygen, cisplatin, mitomycin C, 5-FU, hydroxyurea, bleomycin, paclitaxel, docetaxel, and cetuximab [monoclonal antibody against EGFR (Epidermal Growth Factor Receptor)]

Ans 17:
- a. 4D-CT: (Time being the fourth dimension)
- b. Parathyroid adenoma – pre-operative assessment
- c. Higher radiation doses given

SECTION 8

SKILL ASSESSMENT TOPICS

SECTION OUTLINE

23. Skill Assessment Topics

Skill Assessment Topics

As per the Competency-based Undergraduate Curriculum for the Indian Medical Graduate, the knowledge/skill of each student on a topic may be assessed in various ways as applicable.

LEARNING OBJECTIVES FROM THE COMPETENCIES TABLE AS PER THE COMPETENCY-BASED UNDERGRADUATE CURRICULUM FOR THE INDIAN MEDICAL GRADUATE

K	Knows	A knowledge attribute: Student usually enumerates or describes
KH	Knows How	A higher level of knowledge: Student is able to discuss or analyze
S	Shows	A skill attribute: Student is able to identify or demonstrate the steps
SH	Shows How	A skill attribute: Student is able to interpret/demonstrate a complex procedure requiring thought, knowledge and behavior
P	Performs (under supervision or independently)	Mastery for the level of competence: When done independently or under supervision a prespecified number of times—certification or capacity to perform independently results

The **SUGGESTED ASSESSMENT METHODS** for assessing a student's knowledge in otorhinolaryngology are as follows:
- Written
- Viva voce
- Skill Assessment
- OSCE

Here, we have tried to summarize the topics (**i.e., Competencies**) from the curriculum, for which the suggested assessment method is **"SKILL ASSESSMENT"** or **"OSCE"**.

Students are advised to go through and prepare these topics in a way that they can demonstrate the specific skills involved or perform the examination procedures when asked in the examination.

SKILL ASSESSMENT TOPICS

Clinical Skills

Elicit, document and present an appropriate history in a patient presenting with an **ENT complaint.**

Demonstrate the correct technique of:
1. Use of a **headlamp** in the examination of the ear, nose and throat.
2. Examination of the ear including **otoscopy**.
3. Performance and interpretation of **tuning fork tests**.
4. Examination of the nose and paranasal sinuses including the use of **nasal speculum**.
5. Examining the throat including the use of a **tongue depressor**.
6. Examination of neck including elicitation of **laryngeal crepitus**.
7. Perform and interpret pure tone audiogram and **impedance audiogram**.
8. Choose correctly and interpret radiological, microbiological and histological **investigations** relevant to the ENT disorders.
9. Identify and describe the use of **common instruments used in ENT surgery**.
10. Describe and identify by clinical examination malignant and pre-malignant ENT diseases.
11. Counsel and administer **informed consent** to patients and their families in a simulated environment.
12. Identify, resuscitate and manage **ENT emergencies** in a simulated environment (including tracheostomy, anterior nasal packing, removal of foreign bodies in ear, nose, throat and upper respiratory tract).
13. Demonstrate the correct technique to **instilling topical medications** into the ear, nose and throat in a simulated environment.

Management of Diseases of Ear, Nose and Throat

Elicit, document and present a correct **history**, *demonstrate and describe the* **clinical features**, *choose the correct* **investigations** *and describe the principles of* **management** *of:*

1. Otalgia.
2. Diseases of the external ear.
3. Acute suppurative otitis media (ASOM).
4. Otitis media with effusion (OME).
5. Discharging ear.
6. Chronic suppurative otitis media (CSOM).
7. Squamosal type of CSOM.
8. Hearing loss.
9. Nasal obstruction.
10. Nasal polyps.
11. Adenoids.
12. Allergic rhinitis.
13. Vasomotor rhinitis.
14. Acute and chronic rhinitis.
15. Epistaxis.

16. Acute and chronic sinusitis.
17. Dysphagia.
18. Acute and chronic tonsillitis.
19. Hoarseness of voice.
20. Airway emergencies.
21. Foreign bodies in the air and food passages.
22. Demonstrate the correct technique to hold visualize and **assess** the mobility of the **tympanic membrane** and interpret and diagrammatically represent the findings.
23. Demonstrate the correct technique for **syringing wax from the ear** in a simulated environment.
24. Enumerate the indications and interpret the results of an **audiogram**.

Integration

1. Demonstrate (i) **hearing,** (ii) **testing for smell,** and (iii) **taste sensation** in volunteer/simulated environment.
2. **Counsel patients** to risks of oral cancer with respect to tobacco, smoking, alcohol and other causative factor.
3. Elicit, document and present age appropriate history of a **child with upper respiratory problem** including stridor.
4. Interpret **X-ray of the paranasal sinuses and mastoid**; and/or use written report in case of management.
5. Interpret **CXR in foreign body aspiration and lower respiratory tract infection**, understand the significance of thymic shadow in pediatric chest X-ray.

Bibliography

1. Cummings CW, Flint PW. Cummings's Otolaryngology: Head and Neck Surgery, Seventh edn. Philadelphia PA: Elsevier/Saunders; 2021.
2. Mansour S, Magnan J, Ahmed HH, Nicolas K, Louryan S. Comprehensive and Clinical Anatomy of the Middle Ear. Springer; 2013.
3. Richard LD, Vogl AW, Mitchell WM. Gray's Anatomy for Students, Fourth edn. Philadelphia PA: Elsevier; 2020.
4. Sataloff RT, Hartnick CJ. Sataloff's Comprehensive Textbook of Otolaryngology: Head and Neck Surgery: Pediatric Otolaryngology. Jaypee Brothers Medical Publishers Pvt. Ltd; 2015.
5. Watkinson JC, Clarke R (Eds.). Scott-Brown's Otorhinolaryngology, Head and Neck Surgery, Eighth edn: 3 volumes. CRC Press; 2018.

Bibliography

Index

A

Acoustic neuroma 193
Adenoid 198
Adenoid cystic carcinoma 95
Adenoid facies 104
Adenoid hypertrophy 58, 104
Adenotonsillectomy 192
Airway
    emergencies 199
    management, emergency 110
    obstruction 126
Alcohol consumption 100
Allergic fungal rhinosinusitis 172
Allergic rhinitis 198
Aphthous ulcers 91
Argon tunable dye laser 190
Arnold's nerve 5
Arytenoid cartilage 114
Asch forceps 152
Asch's septal forceps 69
Audiogram 38, 39, 40, 41, 199
    impedance 198
Audio-vestibulometry 37
Auditory canal
    external 3
    internal 9
Auditory placode 36
Auditory vesicle 36
Auerbach's plexus 168
Aural speculum 140
Auricle 4
    development of 31

B

Barium swallow study 102, 160
Beahr's triangle 132
Benign tumor 94
Betel-nut chewing, habit of 87
Bifid uvula 104
Blakesley forceps 152
Blood-stained nasal discharge 63
Body's equilibrium, maintenance of 15
Bone conduction 25
Boyer pre-epiglottic space 114
Boyle Davis mouth gag 153
Brachytherapy 192
Branchial cyst 127
Branchial fistula 168
Branchial sinus 127
Breathing, open-mouth 99
Bronchoscope, rigid 154
Brown adipose tissue 172
Buccal mucosa
    carcinoma, histologic type of 84
    left 84
Bull's eye lamp 140
Butterfly vestibulometry 46

C

Caldwell-Luc operation 56
Candida albicans 92
Carcinoma 177
    in tongue 84
    of maxillary sinus 69
    radiotherapy for 182, 183
Cheek swelling, left sided 161
Chest, digital X-ray 166
Coblator II surgery system 191
Cochlear implant 26
Concave mirror 140
Conductive hearing loss 45
Continuous positive airway pressure 104
Cotton-Myer grading 115
Crico-arytenoid joint 115
Cricothyroid muscle 114
Crocodile forceps 140
Cyberknife 193

D

Debris 19
Delta-aminolevulinic acid 190
Dennis-Browne tonsil holding forceps 153
Diffuse esophageal spasm 104
Dohlman's procedure 103, 166
Double density sign 170, 172
Drooling 159
Dysphagia 98, 102, 162, 199

E

Ear
    canal 19
    discharge 198
        recurrent 20
    examination 136
    external and middle 5, 32

surgery 143, 151
    incisions for 27
    syringing wax 199
Earache, child with 23
Ectoderm 36
Electrolarynx 115
Electromagnetic waves, high-frequency 178
Endobronchial tumors 190
Endoscopic sinus surgery, functional 73
Endotracheal intubation, used for 151
Endotracheal tube 151
ENT
    emergencies 198
    surgery, instruments used in 198
    X-rays in 157
Epiglottis 114
Epistaxis 198
    and nasal mass, history of 67
Esophagoscope, rigid 154
Esophagus 96, 101
Esthesioneuroblastoma, origin of 65
Ethmoid sinus 80
Excision, planning for 65
External beam radio therapy 192
External nose, anatomy of 49

F

Facial swelling, right sided 63
Farabeuf mastoid periosteal elevator 151
Fever, ear discharge with 23
Fiberoptic laryngoscopy 98, 105, 109-111
Fistula 127
    test 26
Fistulogram 168
Foley's catheter 77
Foreign body
    esophagus 166, 167
    in air and food passages 199
    removal of 166
    right bronchus 167
    sensation 98
Fracture nasal bone 166
Freer's double-ended mucoperichondrial elevator 152
Frog face deformity 70
Frontal and ethmoidal sinuses 64
Fronto-ethmoidal mucocele 69
Fuller's bi-valved metallic tracheostomy tube 154

G

Gamma knife 193
Ganglion cells 168
Glossopharyngeal nerve 103

Glottic growth 114
Gluck-Sorenson incision 126
Graves' disease 130
Graves' ophthalmopathy 132
Gurgling sound 98

H

Haemophilus influenzae 25, 166
Hartman's forceps 140
Head and neck cancers 180, 190
Head malignancy 184
Headlamp, use of 198
Hearing aid 26
Hearing, decreased 99
Hearing loss 198
    type of 37
Heller's operation, modified 168
Hematoporphyrin derivative 190
Hemithyroidectomy 132
Hemi-transfixion incision 76
Herpes labialis 92
Heterogeneous signal intensity 172
High-resolution computed tomography 169
Ho's triangle 126
Hoarseness of voice 199
Human papilloma virus 115
Hyperbaric oxygen therapy 191
Hypoglossal nerve palsy 92

I

Image guided radiotherapy treatment 192
Incus-malleus complex 172
Infections, recurrent 33
Inner ear 32, 34
    anatomy of 8
Inspiratory stridor 159
Instilling topical medications 198
Integration 199
Intensity modulated radiotherapy treatment 192

J

Jacobson's nerve 10
Jobson-Horne probe 140
Jugular lymph nodes 127
Juvenile nasopharyngeal angiofibroma 70, 172, 187, 192
Juvenile onset recurrent respiratory papillomatosis 115

K

Kashima operation 192
Killian long-bladed nasal speculum 152

Killian's dehiscence 166
Killian's incision 76
Killian-Jamieson triangle 103
Koerner's septum 36

L

Labyrinth, anatomy of 7
Laimer triangle 103
Laryngeal cancer, advanced 111
Laryngeal crepitus 198
Laryngeal nerve, recurrent 132
Laryngeal papillomas 192
Laryngeal web 114
Laryngopharyngeal cancer 186
Larynx
    and trachea 105
    congenital lesion of 109
    coronal section of 108
    intrinsic muscles of 108
    sagittal section of 107
    squamous cell carcinoma of 171
Laser beam 175
Lempert's endaural
    incision 30
    speculum 151
Leukoplakia 91
Lingual thyroid, suspicion of 129
Lip
    lower, recurrent swelling on 86
    reddish lesion on lateral part of 86
Lower respiratory tract infection 199
Luc's forceps 152
Ludwig's angina 126
Lymphadenopathy 127
Lyre's sign 127

M

MacEwen's triangle 11
Malleus handle, level of 5
Mastoid 199
    air calls 167
    development of 32
    digital X-ray 167
Mastoidectomy, complete 28
Maxilla, frontal process of 167
Maxillary sinus 58, 80, 167
Medial longitudinal fasciculus 16
Mesotympanum 7
Micro laryngeal surgery 115, 176
Microlaryngoscopy 190
Microscope 151
Middle ear anatomy 6
Middle turbinate 77
    anatomy of 54

Mollison self-retaining hemostatic mastoid
    retractor 151
Mondini's dysplasia 36
Moraxella catarrhalis 25
Mouth, right angle of 87
Mucocele 91
Muffled voice 159
Multiple vesicles, clusters of 88
Mylohyoid muscle 95

N

Nasal airflow 57
Nasal bone 54, 167
    digital X-ray 166
Nasal cavity 63, 65
Nasal endoscopic 97
Nasal examination 138
Nasal masses 65
Nasal obstruction 60, 63, 198
    right side 63
Nasal polyps 198
Nasal septal hemangioma 70
Nasal septum 65
    anatomy of 52
    blood supply of 52
Nasal speculum, use of 198
Nasal surgery 145, 152
Nasopharyngeal carcinoma 188
Nasopharynx 103
Neck
    and thyroid, ultrasound of 132
    dissection
        incisions for 123
        types of 122
    examination of 126
    lymph node levels in 119
    malignancy 184
    rapid painful swelling in 121
    spaces 93
Negus knot tier 154
Negus second artery forceps 153
Nose
    and paranasal sinuses 47
    CT scan of 51
    structures on lateral wall of 50

O

Odynophagia, intermittent 102
Ohngren's line 69
Olfactory epithelium 70
Omohyoid muscle 126
Optic nerve 70
Oral cavity 83
    lesions in 88

parts of 85
squamous cell carcinoma of 171
Oral thrush 92
Orbit, causing displacement of 64
Orbital apex syndrome 70
Orbital hematoma 77
Organ of Corti 13
Oropharyngeal surgery 147, 153
Ossicular lever action 17
Osteoradionecrosis 192
Otalgia 198
Otitis media with effusion 30, 198
Otocyst 36
Otosclerosis, surgery for 28
Otoscope 140, 198
  used for 140

P

Palate, embryological development of 78
Paraganglioma 127
Paraglottic space 114
Paranasal sinuses 199
  CT scan of 79
  development of 79
  digital X-ray of 167
Parapharyngeal abscess 103
Parathyroid gland 128
Parotid gland 94
Paterson-Brown Kelly syndrome 104
Pencil-tip sign 166
Peritonsillar abscess 103
Persistent discharging sinus 165
Petro-squamosal suture 36
Pharyngeal pouch 103
Pharynx 96
Photodynamic therapy 190
Photosan-3 190
Pinna 4
Plastic bead 74
Pleomorphic adenoma 95
Plummer-Vinson syndrome 104, 168
Polypoidal nasal mass, unilateral 66
Polyvinyl alcohol particles 194
Positron emission tomography scan 172
Pott's puffy tumor 70
Primitive nose, embryological
    development of 78
Profuse epistaxis, recurrent episodes
    of 170
Proliferative lesion over hard palate 89
Pyramidal process 30

R

Radical neck dissection, modified 126
Radiofrequency ablation device 191

Radiofrequency waves 191
Radiosensitizer agents 194, 188
Radiotherapy setup 184
Ranula 91
Rectus
  lateral 16
  medial 16
Respiratory distress 159
  gradual development of 112
Retropharyngeal abscess 167
Retrotympanum 7
Rhinitis
  acute 198
  chronic 198
Rhinosporidiosis 70
Rhinosporidium seeberi 70
Road traffic accident 62
Robotic surgery 194
Rosen's endomeatal incision 30
Rosenmuller fossa 103

S

Saline-moistened eye pads 190
Salivary gland 94, 93
  neoplasms 89
Schobinger incision 126
Scholastic performance 99
Semi-circular canal 16
  lateral 172
Sensation, burning 90
Sensorineural hearing loss 26
  sudden 191
Septal hematoma 70
Septal swell body 55
Septoplasty 72
  incisions used in 71
Siegel's speculum 140
Sinus
  mucociliary clearance of 56
  plate 167
Sinusitis
  acute 199
  chronic 199
  complications of 64
Skill assessment 197, 198
Skin cancers 190
Smell, testing for 199
Snoring 99
Soft tissue lateral neck, digital X-ray 167
Sound, transmission of 14
Speech development 34
Spinal accessory nerve 126
Squamous cell carcinoma 91
Squamous papilloma 70
St. Clair Thompson adenoid curette with
    cage 154

Stammberger's technique 77
Stapedectomy 30
Steeple sign 166
Stereotactic head frame 193
Stereotactic radiosurgery 184, 188
Streptococcus pneumoniae 25
Stridor 159
Subglottic stenosis 115
Submandibular region 94
Submandibular sialadenitis 95
Submucous cleft palate 104
Substernal chest pain 102
Superficial lobe, enlargement of 94
Superficial ulcers, develops recurrent 85
Superior orbital fissure syndrome 70
Suppurative otitis media
    acute 198
    chronic 198
Supraclavicular fossa 126
Supraomohyoid neck dissection 126
Swallowing, difficulty 160
Swelling
    intermittent 94
    non-tender 64
    on left side of neck 123
    on right side of face 63

T

Taste sensation 199
Tegmen 167
Temporal bone 169
Temporalis fascia graft 30
Thermal repair, zone of 190
Thermoplastic mask 180
Throat
    and intermittent pain 98
    examination 139
    infections, recurrent 97
    surgery 147, 153
Thumb sign 166
Thyroarytenoid muscle 114
Thyroglossal duct cyst 126
Thyroid gland 128
    management of 131
    upper pole of 130
Thyroid imaging reporting and data systems 132
Thyroidectomy 129, 132
Tissue
    ablation 178
    necrosis, zone of 190
Tongue
    base of 129
    depressor 198
    hemangioma of 91
    protrusion of 121, 128
    radiofrequency ablation of 191
    tie 92
    ulcerative lesion on 84
Tonsillar bed 96
Tonsillar dissector 153
Tonsillitis
    acute 199
    chronic 199
Topical sensitizer 190
Touching target tissue 191
Tragus, applying intermittent pressure on 23
Transfixion incision 76
Transilluminant swelling 124
Trauma, history of 157
Trigeminal nerve, ophthalmic division of 70
Trousseau tracheal dilator 154
Tuning fork test 19, 37, 198
Tympanic membrane 14, 21, 199
Tympanogram 40, 42

U

Ulcero-proliferative lesion 84
Uncinate process, types of attachment of 50
Upper respiratory infection
    episode of 41
    fever with 21

V

Vanillylmandelic acid 127
Vasomotor rhinitis 198
Vertigo, complaints of 43
Vestibular nucleus 16
    Vestibule, inflammation of 53
Vestibulo-ocular reflex 18
Vocal abuse 114
Vocal cord
    nodule 114
    position of 109, 115

W

Walsham forceps 152
Water's view 167
Wigand's technique 73, 77

X

Xerostomia 192
Xylometazoline 77

Z

Zenker's diverticulum 103, 166
Zygomatic arch 167